P9-DEJ-249

The Health Care Future

The
Health
Care
Future

James J. Pattee, M.D.
Orlo J. Otteson, M.A.

DEFINING
THE ARGUMENT

HEALING
THE DEBATE

North Ridge Press

© Copyright 1997 James J. Pattee & Orlo J. Otteson

All rights reserved. No portion of this book may be reproduced in any form, except for brief quotations in reviews, without the express written permission of the publishers:

North Ridge Press
17830 Eighth Avenue North
Plymouth, Minnesota 55447

1 888 473 5999

ISBN 1-889279-04-8

Book and jacket design by Will H. Powers
Designed and produced by Stanton Publication Services, Inc.
Saint Paul, Minnesota

Table of Contents

PPR = Beneficience (paternalism)
Autonomy (patient)
utilitarian (quoter)
good / #

77-8 = Market comparison
87-91 = health disparity this

Preface

We began this book in early 1993 – a time when the health care reform discussion had moved to the top of the national agenda. And as we watched the debate intensify, we grew increasingly concerned about the ways certain proposed changes held the potential for creating unanticipated and deleterious effects throughout the entire health care system. Many proposals, in our view, had insufficiently considered the *Law of Unintended Consequences* — and the ways in which changes in one part of the system can produce unforeseen changes in another part.

We concluded that major decisions must take into account system dynamics and their relation to change, and we further concluded that major decisions must also reflect deeply-rooted social and cultural *values*. We thus began our discussion with a brief analysis of values — their nature and function and their role in decision-making. While examining the values issue, we grew interested also in broad justice and social ethics issues — and the ways in which they both reflect our values and influence our health care policy decisions.

With the demise of the Clinton plan and the decline of the health care debate, we reached some general conclusions:

- Much of the reform discussion has been captured by economists, planners, legislators, and other "experts" who have left the broad public "behind in the dust".
- Effective and lasting change requires not only the voices of analysts, experts, and physician leaders from many disciplines—but also the voices and probings of the "lay" public (so-called).
- Most changes will occur at the organizational level and within definable systems across the continuum of care.

These changes, in our view, will be guided by ongoing and persistent inquiry into the fundamental cultural values that underlie and support our health care system. And successful reform efforts will rest heavily on our ability to formulate policies that reflect our basic value and justice concepts. Moreover, continual probing into fundamental values (by experts and "nonexperts" alike) may help loosen the grip of powerful interest groups—and ultimately may ameliorate some of the social dilemmas that obstruct change and innovation.

American society faces large and daunting social problems. The tactics and strategies we develop for addressing health care issues will influence our approaches to other social problems—and may ultimately influence the direction of American culture (Who are we? And what do we wish to become?).

In this brief discussion, we've attempted to define some central (and highly interrelated) philosophical, systemic, and organizational issues that critically affect health care decision-making. We hope the book will illuminate both the complexities and the opportunities that lie ahead. And we hope it will provide a starting place for all citizens ("lay" and professional) to begin developing a broad, value-based dialogue that recognizes interest conflicts and value conflicts—and then finds ways to resolve resultant social dilemmas.

The Health Care Future

1

Health Care Reform
Perspectives, Complexities, and Dilemmas

Our most recent attempt to institute broad health care system reform reminds us again of the various ways competing social values and political ideologies—together with a deep ambivalence toward government-initiated programs—can thwart social change efforts. We've missed another opportunity to develop a fairer and more effective health system. And along the way we've missed yet one more opportunity to launch a wide-open, far-ranging public discussion about the deepest health care questions.

Questions, for example, like these:

What is the meaning of health and what are the goals of medicine in our American society?

We pour enormous resources into a powerful scientific medical model that reacts to illness. But we often fail to consider the benefits and burdens of these interventions—both to individuals and to the broad society. And too frequently we fail to consider all the elements that *produce* physical, psychological, and social health. We've designed a modern health care system dedicated to conquering all illness and disability and staying death's hand. But can

3

health care offer more than the false hope of immortality? And can we identify more clearly the *social context* of health and illness—and then construct social policies that enhance our overall national health status?

What cultural and individual values underlie our health care system, and what value conflicts impede our health reform efforts?
Values represent enduring beliefs, and they guide our policy decisions in powerful and often poorly-understood ways. We seek family security, for example, while simultaneously striving to maintain the fullest degree of freedom, autonomy, and choice. Can we strike some balance between our freedom and our security needs—and then construct health care policies that reflect that balance? Can we identify our existing value hierarchy—and then develop a health care system that incorporates our deeply-ingrained individual, family, social, and cultural values?

What distributive and procedural justice principles underlie our health care system, and what balance among the distributive principles of equity, equality, and need will help us make wiser resource allocation decisions?
Distributive justice principles powerfully shape our health care allocation decisions. But we've yet to define clearly the relation between justice concepts and policy formulations—and to develop effective methods for introducing various (often competing) distributive justice perspectives into our health care policy discussions. Is health care a commodity that we freely exchange in our free market economy according to an *equity* principle—according, that is, to one's investment in the community (in the common social good) and one's ability to pay? Or is it a "special" social good that we distribute *equally* to all citizens. Or should we allocate health care resources solely according to *need*? Or, perhaps, should our allocation system attempt to find some balance (however imperfect) among these three distributive justice principles?

What ethical dilemmas interfere with our ability to formulate more equitable and effective health care policies?

Our health care wants have become needs—and our needs have become rights. But a right to what? And to how much? And for whom? When we define health care as a right, we raise large questions. To what extent is an individual entitled to make a claim on society's resources—and to what extent is society obligated to meet that claim? Can we formulate a medical decision-making process that maintains patient autonomy and physician integrity— while recognizing and contributing to the broad common good?

How do we meet the health care needs of all citizens in the face of finite resources and infinite needs?

Today's economic realities confront us with a harsh truth: we can no longer afford all the health care we desire. Our steadily rising need (real and perceived) for health care—together with medicine's ability to develop processes and technologies that meet those needs—threaten our national economic and social stability. We must find ways to limit our insatiable demand for health care. But are we willing to recognize financial constraints and institute policies that might limit certain forms of care? And are we willing to place constraints on freedoms and behaviors that inflate health care costs?

What is the role of the medical education system in promoting and sustaining systemic, long-term changes in our health care system?

Academic medical centers and medical educators play a central and vital role in formulating and instituting broad health care policies. But many Americans see a growing discontinuity between medical education activities and society's general health needs. And many citizens continue to question whether the medical education establishment is sufficiently and appropriately engaged with the major health care issues of the day. Can the medical education enterprise broaden its perspective and find ways to help society develop a firm primary care foundation?

What new kinds of organizational and leadership models will help us change our health care organizations?
Many (if not most) health care reform measures ultimately will be carried out at the organizational level. But many health care organizations lack the vision, flexibility, and leadership to meet contemporary challenges. What kinds of new "mental models" will help us reshape our health organizations? How can we promote efficiencies and innovations across the continuum of health care? And what kinds of total quality management concepts will help us stimulate organizational change and innovation?

These kinds of questions (and dozens more) perplex us. They're intimidatingly difficult. And they resist firm answers. But they are central and vital—and ultimately unavoidable. Until we address these fundamental (some might say almost existential) questions, our change efforts will continue to bog down in narrow quibbles over policy. Until we understand and confront these deeper health care issues, our attempts to restructure our health care system will falter—and perhaps ultimately fail.

Thus far, our national health care reform discussion has tended to focus on the system's structural deficiencies and venalities: 1) on planning and development strategies that attempt to ensure access, 2) on regulatory strategies that strive to protect consumers' interests, 3) on delivery reorganization strategies that seek to improve efficiency and effectiveness, and 4) on financing and insurance strategies that try to help people buy into the system.

The experts and policy makers who analyze these kinds of issues have seized control of the debate. And our national health care discourse seems trapped in a contentious, acrimonious, arcane policy debate—an argument that most Americans only barely understand and others find irrelevant. Books and journals on health care policy (usually dry as dust) add little to our general understanding. And the political rhetoric at all levels seems designed to increase the confusion, misunderstanding, fear, frustration, scapegoating, and wishful thinking surrounding health policy discussions.

We've focused our attention on narrow health policy issues. And this focus has limited our ability (and our need) to see health care as an ethical and cultural issue—heavily value-laden and tied to our most basic notions of who we are as individuals and what we wish to become as a society.

This book seeks to reframe the national health care discussion. It's directed toward those who wish to think anew and to view health care and health care reform activities in a broader context—away from arguments about payment systems, for example, and toward an examination of the philosophical dilemmas, cultural contradictions, and organizational shortcomings that block change and innovation. We hope the book will help readers see more clearly the interrelated forces that influence our health care system, the basic philosophical conflicts that slow (often defeat) change, and the ways in which new "mental models" will help us create a more responsive and inclusive health system. We hope it will illuminate the health care system's complexity and clarify the central dilemmas that impede health care reform.

The challenge of health care reform

Health care reformers—and those who think about reform—must come to grips with a central question: What kinds of changes can we realistically expect to achieve in our democratic, pluralistic, multiethnic, multiracial, culturally diverse, and religiously variegated American society?

We frequently strive for a master "blueprint" that will save us from piecemeal, middle-of-the-road approaches. And proponents of broad change at the macro level make some strong arguments:

1) Incrementalism, they say, transforms a system gradually by adding new components as the system grows—a viable approach when systems stay relatively simple. When systems grow complex, however, changes in one part may adversely affect other parts—and ultimately defeat change efforts.

2) Moreover, say the macro change proponents, the incremental approach empowers the vested interests. And when participants lack agreement on a long-range plan, all parties demand to be "held harmless" (to suffer no unilateral disadvantage) each step of the way. Thus, the achievable steps tend to be those that *add* immediate advantage to all—not those that require short-term sacrifices in the interest of the long-term common good.

3) In addition, say the broad change advocates, we tend to address problems only when they become serious or obvious enough to move a coalition. And then the coalition moves move only as far as it's compelled to. Consequently, change actions tend to be short-term patchups that fail to loosen the grip of underlying, obstructionist forces.

Thus, say proponents of broad social change (the "anti-incrementalists"), although the health care system evolved incrementally with no overall plan, each evolutionary step was strongly influenced by specific political, social, economic, and professional interests—all of whom gained strength with each step. The health care system, these critics say, may look fragmented and its financing mechanisms may appear incongruent, but the constellation of forces operating within the system give it an inner logic that resists incremental transformations. And only major change at the macro level will produce significant reform.[1]

This argument for broad and bold change holds some validity—and more than a little appeal. We yearn for major "fixes" and broad system changes that will give us a more rational and consistent health care framework. But proposals for sweeping reform fail to consider some basic American cultural and political realities.

First, complex social systems (including the extraordinarily complex health care system) yield slowly to change efforts—when they yield at all. Powerful interests work hard to serve their constituencies—and to preserve the status quo. And many of these special interest groups continue to dominate health care policy formulation.

Second, Americans hold deeply ambivalent attitudes toward government initiatives and publicly-supported social programs. The American public often simultaneously supports *and* opposes government-led reform initiatives. Consequently, both the opponents and supporters of a social policy proposal frequently draw legitimately on competing elements of public opinion. The result? Our political system—already at the mercy of special interests and short-range goals—finds it difficult to develop a vision that will support long-term, broad social change. Lacking a clear consensus about our long-range health care goals, we've often been forced to develop national health policy along the lines of least resistance.

In addition, Americans believe in the dignity, indeed the sacredness, of the individual. And our prevailing connections to individualism frequently limit our ability to formulate collective, broad-scale institutional changes that enhance the common good. Consequently, broad social change in America rarely occurs at the macro level. Social reform in this country tends to find initial support at the grassroots level—and then move forward in incremental steps. The Constitution's checks and balances on political power favor such an approach, and, historically, the approach has served us well in many ways. We've tended to choose middle-ground solutions and to avoid radical, untested new policy directions.

Indeed, our change efforts seem seriously inhibited by our inability even to define clearly our health care goals. What *are* the goals of medicine in American society? What are we trying to accomplish? Can we change our health care system in any meaningful way until we reach some general consensus about its overall mission? And can we reach such a consensus? Our American society—and its health care system—contains so many interconnections and contradictory dynamics that proposed solutions to a social ill often look like attempts to exacerbate the problem.

Moreover, change proponents, including health care providers and consumers, are increasingly called upon to balance their "own" interests with the interests of the community and the society-at-large. This "common good" perspective requires the ability to see 1) the interrelatedness of biological, psychological, social, economic, and political systems in the social environment and 2) the connection between the social environment and the health of individuals. And it asks all citizens to distinguish between the traditional *medical* model and a new *health* model of social change that attempts to place health and illness within a social context. Let's look briefly at the new health care model and its role in our complex health care future.

Health care model vs. medical care model

Medical care focuses on a defined and limited set of symptoms and illnesses that require prevention, treatment, rehabilitation, or maintenance measures—or some combination of these approaches. And practitioners within the medical care (or disease care) model attempt to isolate problems and to advance their inquiry through the use of particularistic and discrete methodologies. The medical care model dominates health care planning and delivery decisions, and our faith in the model has given us a powerful "medical industrial complex" that strongly influences health care policies. But some analysts think that medical care treatment activities—the "care and cure" branch of the medical enterprise—influence only about one-quarter to one-third of all health status. The other two-thirds to three-quarters, they say, are influenced by broad (and interdependent) biological, psychological, social, and spiritual *health care* factors.[2]

Over the years, the traditional medical model has steadily broadened the definitions of health and illness, and Americans have looked strongly to the model for help in treating family, social, and economic "illnesses" (alcoholism, poverty, and child abuse, for example) The victims of these social pathologies bring long-standing medical and developmental problems into the medical care system—problems that frustrate and burden the scientific and technologically oriented medical care model.

In recent years, however, a more inclusive *health care* paradigm has begun to challenge the *medical care model's* grip on health planning and policy-making activities. This new "systems approach" holds that our health system change efforts have been stalled by reactive and particularistic approaches—and by outdated and ineffective "mental models" (deeply ingrained assumptions, even images) that foster institutional torpor. The new paradigm attempts to 1) map the continuous, dynamic interrelationships among and between various political and social factors, values concepts, and health policy issues and then 2) develop an intervention philosophy that rests less on concepts of control and more on "inquiring systems"—on systems that continually learn and proactively seek ways to develop "alternative realities."[3]

Our medical care system continues to make enormous contributions to individual health, and we must continue to develop the medical model's best features. Some recent empirical studies, however, show strong causal relations between individuals' health status and certain social factors—income and education levels, for example. And future health status advances will rest heavily on our ability to understand the *social context of health*—and then to formulate broad national policies that address the social determinants of health.

Whither health care?

Given all the political, philosophical, economic, cultural, and organizational impediments to social change, how can we develop a health care system that fairly distributes care and shares burdens? How can we temper the influence of scientific medicine and find a balance between the medical and health care models? How can we reduce the tension between our wish for health security and our insistence on freedom and autonomy—and then find some balance among the distributive justice principles of equity, equality, and need? And how can we develop new mental models about 1) the ways in which individuals and groups relate to each other within health care organizations and 2) the ways in which those organizations relate to each other across the continuum of health care?

We needn't wait for crisis to turn into chaos before we launch a *change process* that will begin to ameliorate seemingly intractable conflicts and dilemmas. But if broad institutional reform seems out of reach for now, where then do we begin? How should we commence?

First, we must recognize that micro-innovations at the intraorganizational and inter-organizational level can join with macrochanges at the institutional and societal level to produce meaningful transformations. And we must recognize that "breakthrough" changes often reflect the interplay of smaller changes that build slowly over time and combine to create new institutional systems and paradigms. James Brian Quinn calls this process *logical incrementalism* and describes it this way:

The most effective strategies of major enterprises tend to emerge step-by-step from an iterative process in which the organization probes the future, experiments, and learns from a series of partial (incremental) commitments rather than through global formulations of total strategies. Good managers are aware of this process, and they consciously intervene in it. They use it to improve the information available for decisions and to build the psychological identification essential to successful strategies. The process is both logical and incremental. Such logical incrementalism is not "muddling," as most people understand that word. Properly managed, it is a conscious, purposeful, proactive, executive practice. Logical incrementalism honors and utilizes the global analyses inherent in formal strategy formulation models. It also embraces the central tenets of the political or power-behavioral approaches to such decision-making. But it does not become subservient to any one model. Instead each approach becomes simply a component in a logical process that improves the quality of available information, establishes critical elements of political power and credibility, creates needed participation and psychological commitment, and thus enhances both the quality of strategic decisions and the likelihood of their successful implementation.[4]

We must continue to push for macro changes at the state and national levels—changes in reimbursement systems, for example. But changes at the macro levels come slowly and are driven by powerful social, economic, and political forces that often seem beyond our reach. And many of these forces possess interests and agendas (often hidden) that confuse the dialogue and hold the potential for undermining the common social good. Major structural health care reform moves slowly, and inherent social and cultural contradictions often obstruct any meaningful change. But if we can join major structural changes with micro-innovations at the community and organizational level—and then institute effective processes of inquiry and change *across the continuum of health care*—we may achieve surprising results.

Purpose and nature of the book

The health care system can be studied and analyzed from many different distances, altitudes, and angles. We've chosen to address some basic—but seldom-discussed—issues that powerfully influence (often unconsciously) our health care policy decisions. And we hope our discussions will promote a more logical, rational, and useful public discourse. We've included suggested readings at the end of each chapter for readers who wish to broaden their knowledge about specific issues.

Here's a brief preview of the book's topics. The book divides into three main sections.

The first section addresses some fundamental moral philosophical issues:

Chapter 1. Introduction. Whither health care?

Chapter 2. Health care and the nature of values. What are individual and social values? And why do we need to understand health care change within the context of a value system?

Chapter 3. Health care and the idea of justice. What is distributive and procedural justice? And what is their relevance to health care resource allocation decisions?

Chapter 4. Health care and ethics. What ethical dilemmas limit our ability to formulate politically feasible and culturally acceptable health care policies? How can we find a balance between individual needs and the requirements of the common social good?

Chapter 5. Health care and economics. What forces really drive ballooning health care costs? Can we contain those costs? What's the relation between medical ethics and health economics?

The second section addresses specific issues in health care organizational life:

Chapter 6. Health care quality and organizational life. How can health care organizations effectively meet the simultaneous requirements of efficiency and quality? What is the continuous quality improvement concept, and what's its value to a health care quality management system?

Chapter 7. Health care and the Deming management method. How can W. Edwards Deming's perspectives and Fourteen Points help health care organizations develop continuous quality improvement strategies?

Chapter 8. Health care and the "learning organization?" How can Peter Senge's concepts help health care organizations develop new mental models and a new vision?

Chapter 9. Health care and systems thinking. What is systems thinking? How can it help us see the "big picture" and address organizational complexities more effectively?

Chapter 10. Health care and leadership. How do leaders and managers differ? And what new leadership model will most effectively serve the modern health care organization?

The third section describes some new perspectives that will carry us into our complex future:

Chapter 11. Health care and the medical education system. What role does medical education play in health care reform efforts? And how can the "population perspective" better meet society's health care needs?

Chapter 12. Conclusion. What new vision will help us overcome tenacious assumptions and move us toward more effective health care models and interventions?

Conclusion

In 701 B.C. a small community within the walled city of Jerusalem found itself under siege by a powerful and steadily-advancing Assyrian army. The Assyrians demanded an immediate surrender, and behind the walls the besieged community members gathered to discuss their options and possibilities. Armed with new visions, they approached the wall and through a common language established a dialogue with the enemy. The resultant dialogue transformed perceptions on both sides, and the hostilities ceased. The conversation "at the wall" helped both those "behind the wall" and those "outside the wall" create tools for listening and seeing— and for expanding their imaginations.

The national health care discussion, in our view, must find ways to move its "internal discourses" and "external discourses" to the wall—and then resolve problems and create opportunities through "conversations at the wall."

Social problems cannot be solved by the disciplined and professional pursuit of abstract knowledge alone. Indeed, social ills cannot be solved at all—in the usual sense of being "solved." We will never wholly "fix" our health care system—not now, not ever. We can, however, strive to construct a self-guided society that relentlessly probes and examines social maladies and finds innovative and multifaceted ways to address them. We can establish a process of inquiry and dialogue that will help us 1) define the critical issues, 2) ask the right questions, 3) gather and analyze the relevant data, 4) take appropriate actions, and 5) assess and reevaluate decisions. We hope this book will provide some analytic tools for assisting that process—and for establishing useful and stimulating health care "conversations at the wall."

REFERENCES

1. Alfred Miller and Maria Miller, *Options for Health and Health Care: The Coming of Post-Clinical Medicine* (New York: John Wiley & Sons, 1972), 43–57.
2. Leonard Duhl, *Health Planning and Social Change* (New York: Human Sciences Press, 1986), 39.
3. Ibid., 32–47.
4. James Brian Quinn, *Strategies for Change: Logical Incrementalism* (Homewood IL: Irwin, 1980), 58.

SUGGESTED READINGS

Paul Starr, *The Social Transformation of American Medicine* (New York: Basic Books, 1982).

Leonard Duhl, *Health Planning and Social Change* (New York: Human Sciences Press, 1986).

R. R. Alford, *Health Care Politics: Ideological and Interest Group Barriers To Reform* (Chicago: University of Chicago Press, 1975).

Sharon Kaufman, *The Healer's Tale: Transforming Medicine and Culture* (Madison: University of Wisconsin Press, 1993).

Robert Bellah et al., *The Good Society* (New York: Vintage Books, 1991).

2

Values and Health Care Decision-Making

The American health care discussion revolves in many ways around values—around the ends we strive to attain and the means we choose to achieve them. Our actions mainly bespeak our values. *And health care decisions are heavily value-laden.* Our success in reconstituting our health care system will rest heavily on our ability to identify our most deeply-held individual, social, and cultural values—and then construct broad social and health care policies that reflect those values. But what are values? And what's their relation to health care?

What is a value?

A value is an enduring belief that a specific *end-state of existence* (security, freedom) or *mode of conduct* (honesty, competence) is personally or socially *preferable* to another end-state or mode of conduct. Values powerfully shape and guide our private and public lives. They tell us what's right, good, and desirable; and they help us evaluate the morality of our behavior and the degree of our competence. And *value-focused thinking*—the ability to recognize and articulate essential values—lies at the heart of wise social policy decision-making.

But we often view values as private, subjective attitudes— unworthy of serious examination and easily dismissed. "After all," we say to someone with whom we disagree, "that's just your value judgment." Moreover, we periodically reorder our values, and, in the face of disagreement and competing values, we may abandon the quest to identify shared values. We conclude that values are mushy and ill-defined—interesting but difficult to locate and label, and lacking the inherent worth of science-based knowledge.

But we needn't view values as purely subjective phenomena toward which we assume a merely passive, receptive stance. Personal and social values are real and enduring—and, for better or worse, they shape our institutions and direct our life courses in powerful ways. In Moliere's play *Le Bourgeois Gentilhomme*, the character M. Jourdain makes the remarkable discovery that he has been speaking prose all his life—but without knowing it. Similarly, we establish and act on values throughout our lives— but with little conscious awareness. Values powerfully influence our thoughts, feelings, and actions—and they shape our social attitudes, ideologies, and behaviors in important ways. Values underlie our social institutions, and values undergird our complex and critical health care system. But we've yet to reach a firm definition of values. And we've yet to find effective ways of incorporating a values discussion into the national health care dialogue.

End-state of existence and mode of conduct values

Our behavior is influenced by specific personal preferences (needs and desires), specific prescriptions for behavior (shoulds and oughts), general preferences (likes and interests), and general philosophies (morals and ethics). But it's our values that mainly guide our ongoing activities and our *conceptions of the desirable*—both the desirable *end-states of existence* we wish to achieve and the preferable *modes of conduct* we choose to achieve them.

Some individuals attach great importance to individual values and pursue end-states such as personal achievement and comfort. Others (social reformers, for example) emphasize social values and promote end-states such as social justice and broad economic opportunity. We possess far fewer end-state of existence values than mode of conduct values. There are just so many end-states toward which to strive (perhaps a dozen and a half). There are substantially more modes of conduct (perhaps five or six dozen) we can use to attain our desired end-states.[1]

Although individuals and societies possess relatively few values, these values can be arranged in ways that create myriad combinations of value hierarchies. And all the different combinations account for the seemingly endless variation in attitudes and behaviors within and among individuals, organizations, institutions, and societies. A mere eighteen end-state values arranged in order of importance in eighteen factorial ways, can result in 640 trillion variations. Given all the various ways individuals can rank differing values, it's little wonder people react so differently to specific circumstances—and still less a wonder they fail to resolve conflicts and reach consensus on social policy issues.

Milton Rokeach, a values scholar, has noted the "oughtness" of end-state and mode of conduct values. This "oughtness" relates more to mode of conduct values that concern morality. An individual, for example, may feel more societal pressure to behave honestly and responsibly than to behave competently and logically. He or she may feel more pressure to behave morally than to seek individual end-states such as wisdom and happiness.

But the more widely a value is shared throughout society, the greater the degree of "oughtness" we experience. This "ought-

ness" transcends any one individual's point of view and demands
that we all behave in certain ways that benefit others (or at least
doesn't harm them). Any attempts to form a consensus about the
shape of our health care system must take into account our
"oughtness"—our sense of the moral values American society
feels compelled to uphold.[2]

Rokeach goes on to note that the *value concept* occupies a
central position across all the social sciences—sociology, anthro-
pology, psychology, political science, education, economics, history. And, more than any other concept, it holds the potential
for *unifying* the diverse interests of *all* the sciences that address
human behavior. Health care, too, cuts across various disciplines, and we can benefit in many ways by using the value concept to analyze, interpret, and unify the diverse interests that
comprise the health care system—from the individual at the
micro level to the societal and cultural institutions at the macro
level. The value concept is central to the health care discussion
throughout this book, and we will return to it repeatedly in our
later discussions.

What are value systems?

A value possesses a *content* attribute and an *intensity* attribute.
We identify specific values—but we also assign importance to
each. And we organize our values into a *value hierarchy* that
helps us choose between and among possible courses of action.
We weigh our individual and social values against each other and
rank them. We prioritize our values and order them into a value
system that is best understood in terms of a *value hierarchy*. And
this hierarchical concept helps us understand that individuals, organizations, and societies can (indeed must) be viewed not only in
terms of specific values but also in terms of their value *priorities*.

A value system develops bit by bit over the course of a lifetime
and is intricately interwoven with habitual conduct as well as

with more cogitative decision-making activities. The value system is a comprehensive mental structure and matrix that we never fully activate at any one time. We consult the most immediately relevant part and ignore for the moment the rest. We activate different subsets of the system according to the social circumstances in which we find ourselves—and according to the ways in which we have ranked our individual and social values.

The enduring and flexible nature of the value hierarchy

The total value system remains sufficiently stable over time to provide us with some sense of continuity and meaning. But the system also retains the flexibility required to rearrange the hierarchy as changes occur in our personal, family, organizational, community, and societal worlds. Thus, a value system maintains its enduring and stable nature while also preserving its fluid and dynamic qualities.

We reorder our values slowly and reluctantly, but we *can* and *do* reorder them. If our values were completely stable, individual and social change would come too slowly—if at all. If they were completely unstable, we would fail to achieve social order and continuity in human affairs. But we do *prioritize* our values—we rank them in a hierarchical order. And those priorities express themselves in the choices we make and the actions we take. Although our individual values change (up or down in the heirarchy) over time, we seldom make major changes in the entire value system.

Thus, we find that certain values dominate and characterize us. We learn (albeit imperfectly) to reorder certain values in order to cope more effectively with increasingly complex personal, family, community, and societal issues. *And we learn that change—at both the personal and societal levels—depends in large part on our ability to reorder our priorities while maintaining some sense of continuity and meaning.*

The Rokeach Value Survey

Milton Rokeach has identified some central end-state and mode of conduct values. The Rokeach Value Survey, a landmark study, measured American citizens' values four different times—in 1968, 1971, 1974, and 1981. The survey results, shown in Table 1 (facing page), offer a starting point 1) for defining the core values that underlie our present system and 2) for identifying some values that might support a restructured health care system.[3]

These surveys provide insights into the enduring values Americans hold highest. The stability of the values is impressive. The six items that ranked highest in 1981 are identical to the six top-ranked items in 1968 and not one of the six items varies by more than one rank from its 1981 position in any of the three previous surveys (1968, 1971, 1974). The stability of the six lowest-ranking items is almost as impressive. The six lowest-ranked items in the 1981 survey are identical to the six lowest-ranked items in the 1968 survey. And most of the 1981 items do not vary by more than one rank from the items in any of the three previous surveys. Although the six middle items show greater volatility than the top or bottom six, they remain within the middle zone almost without exception. A brief examination of two top values—*family security* and *freedom*—may yield some clues to the main goals (the main end-states of existence) toward which our health care system should strive.

Family security and freedom

Americans value *family security*. Survey respondents ranked family security (defined as the ability to take care of loved ones) first or second in all four polls. Most Americans seem to want a secure environment, adequate and available health care services, and some assurance that catastrophic illness or injury will not wipe them out and destroy the family unit.

24

TABLE 1

Average Rankings of 18 Terminal and 18 Instrumental Values
by Four National Samples of Americans in 1968, 1971, 1974, and 1981

Terminal (End-State) Values	1968	1971	1974	1981
A world at peace (free of war and conflict)	1	1	2	2
Family security (taking care of loved ones)	2	2	1	1
Freedom (independence, free choice)	3	3	3	3
Happiness (contentment)	4	6	5	5
Self-respect (self-esteem)	5	5	4	4
Wisdom (mature understanding of life)	6	7	6	6
Equality (brotherhood, equal opportunity for all)	7	4	12	12
Salvation (being saved, eternal life)	8	9	10	9
A comfortable life (a prosperous life)	9	13	8	8
A sense of accomplishment (lasting contribution)	10	11	7	7
True friendship (close companionship)	11	10	9	10
National security (protection from attack)	12	8	13	11
Inner harmony (freedom from inner conflict)	13	12	11	13
Mature love (sexual and spiritual intimacy)	14	14	14	14
A world of beauty (beauty of nature and the arts)	15	15	15	16
Social recognition (respect, admiration)	16	17	18	18
Pleasure (an enjoyable leisurely life)	17	16	16	17
An exciting life (a stimulating, active life)	18	18	17	15

Instrumental (Mode of Conduct) Values	1968	1971	1974	1981
Honest (sincere, truthful)	1	1		
Ambitious (hardworking, aspiring)	2	3		
Responsible (dependable, reliable)	3	2		
Forgiving (willing to pardon others	4	4		
Broadminded (open minded)	5	5		
Courageous (standing up for beliefs)	6	5		
Helpful (working for welfare of others)	7	7		
Clean (neat, tidy)	8	10		
Capable (Competent, effective)	9	9		
Self-controlled (restrained, self-disciplined	10	11		
Loving (affectionate, tender)	11	8		
Cheerful (lighthearted, joyful)	12	13		
Independent (self-reliant, self-sufficient)	13	12		
Polite (courteous, well-mannered)	14	14		
Intellectual (intelligent, reflective)	15	15		
Obedient (dutiful, respectful)	16	16		
Logical (consistent, rational)	17	17		
Imaginative (daring, creative)	18	18		

Note: Data are from representative national samples of adult Americans by the National Opinion Research Center, University of Chicago, in 1968 (N = 1,409) and 1971 (N = 1,430; see Rokeach, 1974), and by two-wave panel survey (N = 933) by the Survey Research Center, University of Michigan, in 1974 and 1981 (see Inglehart, 1985).

The same survey shows, however, that Americans value highly their *freedom* and *independence*—their right to make free choices. Freedom ranked third in all four polls. American health care consumers, in our view, want the freedom to choose their caregivers and to make informed decisions about their care. In turn, health care providers seek to maintain their integrity and to practice their professions effectively and freely.

Thus, policy makers and legislators struggle to find a formula that will provide patients and providers some form of "health security" for all citizens, while preserving their independence and autonomy. But does the value we attach to family security conflict with our desire for autonomy and freedom? Can we maintain our family security *and* our faith in individualism. Or are we trapped in a *values dilemma*?

These questions help illustrate the *competing* nature of values. The American value system contains sets of contradictory (and partially contradictory) commitments. Values compete and conflict, and the dialectic between and among them adds an element of constant tension to our social change efforts. Many of our lawmakers and policymakers tend to frame value differences and conflicts in terms of "good" versus "bad"—and they often strive to overpower and eliminate opposing values. But value conflicts can be viewed as a positive element that steers us away from simplistic singularity and toward other new perspectives. The presence of conflicting values can serve as a generative force for change. And our expressed wish (as revealed in the Rokeach Value Survey) for both freedom and family security illustrate the need to identify conflicting values and to consider various views in our social policy formulations.

Values and needs

Clashes and conflicts constantly occur among needs—and hence among values. And some theorists, including the late Abraham

Maslow, have attempted to equate values with needs. Needs and values, however, differ significantly. But let's look first at the ways three experts have defined the term *needs*.

Maslow saw a hierarchy of five needs that includes in ascending order 1) physiological needs, 2) safety needs, 3) love needs, 2) esteem needs, and 5) self-actualization needs. Physiological needs, said Maslow, must be addressed before we consider safety needs. Safety needs must be addressed before we consider love needs—and so on. Higher order needs (love, esteem, and self-actualization concerns), according to Maslow, are satisfied internally. Lower order needs (physiological and safety concerns) are satisfied externally.[4]

Clayton Alderfer has used empirical research to rework Maslow's need hierarchy. His *ERG theory* sees three groups of core needs—existence, relatedness, and growth (thus the ERG label). The existence group provides our basic material existence requirements (Maslow's physiological and safety needs). The relatedness group satisfies the desire for important interpersonal relationships. And the growth group fulfills the intrinsic desire for personal development. Unlike Maslow, who saw a rigid steplike progression through the needs, Alderfer thinks 1) that more than one need may be operative at the same time and 2) that if the gratification of a higher-level need is stifled, the desire to satisfy a lower-level need increases.[5]

David McClelland sees three needs: 1) the need for *achievement*—the drive to excel and to achieve in relation to a set of standards; 2) the need for *power*—the ability to manage one's self and to influence others; and 3) the need for *affiliation*—the desire for friendly and close interpersonal relationships.[6]

It's tempting to equate values with needs. But values are more central than needs, and they represent one of our most distinguishing human characteristics. *Values are the cognitive representation and transformation of needs—not only of individual needs but also of societal and institutional demands. Values are the joint results of sociological as well as psychological forces acting upon the individual.* And, in the words of Milton Rokeach, "Once such demands and needs become cognitively transformed into values, they are capable of being defended, justified, advocated, and exhorted as personally and socially desirable."

Rokeach goes on to say:

> Needs may or may not be denied, depending on whether they can stand conscious personal and social scrutiny, but values need never be denied. Thus when a person tells us about his values, he is surely also telling us about his needs. But we must be cautious in how we infer needs from values because values are not isomorphic [possessing a similar structure] with needs. Needs are cognitively transformed into values so that a person can end up smelling himself, and being smelled by others, like a rose.[7]

Our individual health care needs vary from time to time and change gradually (sometimes not so gradually) over time. These changing needs often force changes in our value hierarchy. Individuals, for example, with few health care needs may place a high priority on freedom and choice—and a lesser priority on family health security. Families with high health care needs may place a high priority on family health security—and a lesser priority on individual autonomy.

Individuals with similar health needs often form special interest groups and attempt to change the social value hierarchy in ways that help them meet their needs. Thus, our health care system finds itself buffeted not only by conflicting *values* but also by the competing *needs* and *interests* of various groups. Can we meet every "health" need and interest? Or must we begin to make choices among competing health needs and interests within the context of an explicitly defined value system?

Values and thinking styles

Our difficulties in constructing an understandable, explicit health care value hierarchy are further complicated by the various ways we arrive at our values. Hunter Lewis describes six thinking styles that shape our individual values and influence our social beliefs:[8]

1) *Authority*	We take someone else's word (our parents, for example) or we place our faith in an external authority such as the state. ("I believe in the authority of—")
2) *Deductive logic*	We subject our beliefs to deductive reasoning. ("Since A is true, B must be true.")
3) *Sense experience*	We gain direct knowledge through our five senses. ("I know this is true because I saw it, I heard it, I smelled it, or I touched it myself.")
4) *Emotion*	We feel that something is right. Although we do not usually associate feeling with thinking or judging, we actually "think" and "judge" through our emotions all the time. ("I feel that this is true.")
5) *Intuition*	We use our unconscious-intuitive mind to derive insights and problem solutions. ("When I awoke the next morning, the solution came to me in a flash.")
6) *Science*	We use sense experience to collect the observable facts, intuition to develop a testable hypothesis about the facts, logic to develop the test or experiment, and sense experience again to complete the test. ("I tested the hypothesis experimentally and found that it was true.")

We seldom focus consciously on these six modes of reasoning or thinking styles, but the main point seems clear: *our values are closely related to the way we arrive at them.* By adopting and emphasizing one thinking style over another, we turn it into a dominant personal or social value that colors all other value choices. We say, for example, that the testimony of an authority (e.g., the Bible or the U.S. Constitution) is more *valuable* than the testimony of the emotions, or that the testimony of deductive logic is more *valuable* than the testimony of sense experience—and so on.

If we emphasize one thinking style over another, will that lead us directly to specific social beliefs and actions? Not directly. Individuals and societies rarely rely on a single reasoning mode or thinking style. Rather, they rely on a combination of styles—each with sharply different emphases. And that's one reason human and social values are so subtle, complex, and diverse—and one of several reasons values are so complicated.

Social and cultural values

We've thus far discussed values mainly in terms of individual values. But we also possess *social* and *cultural* values that guide our ongoing activities and shape our institutions. Western values, especially American values, are rooted in

1) the *rationalist tradition*, which holds the intellect supreme, considers humans as conscious and discriminating, and views affective or feeling responses with skepticism;

2) the *Judeo-Christian ethic*, which holds that humans and the universe are endowed with ultimate purpose;

3) the *Anglo-Saxon tradition*, which, joining hands with the rational and religious traditions, extols individualism, holds liberty and equality to be self-evident truths, and espouses the right and ability of people to govern themselves;

4) and the *pragmatic faith*, which holds that the combined rational, religious, and political base (formed over several centuries) is a sound foundation—or at least a sounder one than those formed by most other political and religious groups.[9]

Out of these various sources have come certain "reasons" (to use the American psychiatrist Harry Stack Sullivan's term) that have sunk so deeply into our individual selves we only faintly perceive them. These "reasons," which the sociologist Robert Bellah terms "habits of the heart" and the theologian Richard McCormick calls "value variables," constitute the unwitting aspect of a culture. They exert greater influence on the culture's tone and direction than explicit laws and policies. *And these cultural assumptions, trends, unexamined attitudes, and biases greatly determine the ways we order our cultural values system and heavily influence the ways we think about social issues.*

But can we identify an American cultural value hierarchy? In our pluralistic society, can we define a consistent and integrated cultural value hierarchy and then construct public policies that reflect these values? Can we identify an American "character" or "creed" that will help us reshape our health care system?

Unfortunately, sociologists, cultural historians, and other scholars and analysts still struggle to find a neatly unified national "ethos" or an irresistible "strain toward consistency." We can identify clusters of American *traits* and *attitudes* and *interests* and *social norms. But we have yet to pin down an empirically-tested hierarchy of American social and cultural values. Our pluralistic American society has yet to identify a set of desired end-states and preferable modes of conduct that can form the basis for a viable national health care policy.*

Individualism and the common good

American individualism—the insistence on self-reliance and the emphasis on the importance and independence of the individual—permeates American culture. And some cultural historians think it's the only American cultural value we can identify with any certainty. Alexis de Toucqueville in his classic 1840 study *Democracy in America* defined individualism thus:

> Individualism is a novel expression, to which a novel idea has given birth. Our fathers were only acquainted with egotism. Egotism is a passionate and exaggerated love of self, which leads a man to connect everything with his own person and to prefer himself to everything in the world. Individualism is a mature and calm feeling, which disposes each member of the community to sever himself from the mass of his fellow creatures: and to draw apart with his family and friends: so that, after he has thus formed a little circle of his own, he willingly leaves society at large to itself. . . . Individualism is of democratic origin, and it threatens to spread in the same ratio as the equality of conditions.[10]

We cannot abandon our individualism—nor should we. Our deepest individual and national aspirations and identities are rooted in our sense of individualism. But some of our deepest social problems are linked closely also to our excessive individualism and our claims to unbridled freedom. Excessive individualism has limited our ability to understand the value of broad, community-oriented conceptions of the common good, and it has promoted certain forms of unbridled freedom (freedom without limits and moral commitment) that threaten both our individuality and our sense of shared purpose. *Thus, individualism that passes the contemporary social test emerges as freedom within limits and freedom with a built-in social commitment.*

In recent years, a new politics of citizenship has begun to challenge the centrality of rampant individualism disconnected from societal obligation. A new group of scholars and activists seeks compromises between the arguments of the hard political right and the hard political left. These activists promote *reciprocal obligation*—a community ethic that calls on citizens to balance individual rights with social responsibilities. And their understanding of social justice revolves around the concept of *reciprocity*.

This reciprocal view of society holds that each member of the community owes something to all the rest, and the community owes something to each of its members. Justice, in this view, requires the presence of responsible individuals in a responsive community contributing to the common good. Community members have a responsibility to provide (as well as they can) for themselves and their families. And the community in turn is responsible for protecting each citizen against catastrophe, for ensuring the basic needs of all who genuinely cannot provide for themselves, and for safeguarding a zone within which individuals may define their own lives through free exchange and choice.[11]

In health care, the realization of the common good presupposes initiatives from all sectors of society, including health care providers, purchasers, payers, and institutions. Participation in the common good implies a moral commitment to create constructive forms of social, political, and economic interdependence—*and to find some balance between an individual-centered and a community-centered view of health and human welfare.*

In an increasingly complex, interdependent society and world, much of our success will depend on our willingness and ability to temper our individualism and accommodate it to the worth and needs of others. We cannot escape our prevailing connections to traditional concepts of individualism. But our health care reform efforts can (and must) recognize the ways in which our individualism interferes with our attempts to construct cooperative and inclusive social arrangements.

Values and health care reform

In his book *Value-Focused Thinking*, Ralph L. Keeney describes some ways to identify decision opportunities and to create better alternatives through first recognizing and articulating fundamental *values*. In conventional decision-making, says Keeney, we usually identify alternatives and then choose between or among them. But in value-focused thinking, decision makers first define their end-state of existence values (their goals) and then determine their mode of conduct values—the means that will help them attain their objectives. Since values are more fundamental to a "decision problem," an early and deep focus on values in the decision making process will lead to more desirable consequences—and even to more appealing problems.

When we participate in value-focused thinking, we free ourselves from constraints—from the need to choose between and among lists of prespecified problems or alternatives. Value-focused thinking recognizes that we can *create* alternatives, and that by first defining and focusing on our *values* (both end-state and mode of conduct values), we begin to think in terms of *decision opportunities*—rather than *decision problems*. We bring our values heirarchy to consciousness, and we begin using our values to frame questions, to gather and analyze relevant information, and to form conclusions based on sound logic, reasoned judgments, and carefully acquired data.[12]

The American health care discussion is first of all a debate about values. True and lasting change will require the intelligence and honesty to weigh and know our values—and the creativity and courage to make decisions that reflect those values. True reform will also require a reasoned public discourse that recognizes the role of values in clarifying public policy choices and defining the foundations of a fair, effective health care system.

REFERENCES

1. Milton Rokeach, *The Nature of Human Values* (New York: The Free Press, 1983), 11.
2. Ibid., 9.
3. Milton Rokeach and Sandra J. Ball Rokeach, "Stability and Change in American Value Priorities," *American Psychologist* 44 (May 1989), 775–84.
4. Abraham Maslow, *Motivation and Personality* (New York: Harper & Row, 1954).
5. Clayton Alderfer, "An Empirical Test of a New Theory of Human Needs," *Organizational Behavior and Human Performance* 4 (May 1969): 142–75.
6. David McClelland, *The Achieving Society* (New York: Van Nostrand Reinhold, 1961).
7. Rokeach, *The Nature of Human Values,* 20.
8. Hunter Lewis, *A Question of Values* (New York: HarperCollins, 1990), 5–20.
9. Gail Inlow, *Values in Transition: A Handbook* (New York: John Wiley & Sons, 1972), 1938.
10. Alexis de Tocqueville, *Democracy in America,* trans. George Lawrence, ed. J.P. Mayer (New York: Doubleday, Anchor Books, 1969).
11. Amitai Etzioni, *The Spirit of Community: Rights, Responsibilities, and the Communitarian Agenda* (New York, Crown Publishers, 1993).
12. Ralph Keeney, *Value-Focused Thinking* (Cambridge MA, Harvard University Press, 1992), 3–28.

SUGGESTED READINGS

Hunter Lewis, *A Question of Values* (New York: HarperCollins, 1990).

Milton Rokeach, *The Nature of Human Values* (New York: The Free Press, 1983).

Ralph Keeney, *Value-Focused Thinking* (Cambridge MA: Harvard University Press, 1992).

Robert Bellah et al., *Habits of the Heart* (New York: Harper & Row, 1985).

Reinhard Priester, *Taking Values Seriously: A Values Framework for the U.S. Health Care System* (Minneapolis: University of Minnesota Center for Biomedical Ethics, 1992).

3

Health Care and Distributive Justice:
Balancing Claims of Equality, Equity, and Need

Health care reform discussions lead inevitably to the oldest problem in political philosophy—the nature of justice in a society. Justice issues pervade social life. And *distributive justice principles* influence our most basic health care resource allocation decisions. In an age of competition for social resources and wide public resistance (if not hostility) to more tax-supported social programs, we face fundamental questions. Who gets what—and how much? Who decides? What's fair? Do we allocate health care services equally to all citizens? Or according to need? Or ability to pay? Or according to the requirements of the common good?

These questions puzzle us. We long for a just social order and a fair distribution of health care resources. But in our pluralistic, competitive American society, we rarely (if ever) find an allocation formula that satisfies all groups. Distributive justice principles clash and conflict. And we struggle to strike a balance between and among competing principles that will promote fairer and more effective health care policies.

The idea "each according to his or her needs," for example, begs some central questions. Are the needs perceived or real? Which needs merit our primary consideration? Which needs can we ignore? All sorts of values enter into a definition of needs—and of equity and equality. And all sorts of values enter into—often overpower—our attempts to discuss rationally (and calmly) society's health care resource allocation issues.

Distributive justice principles—explicit and implicit, stated and unstated—powerfully shape our health care allocation decisions. We can't avoid difficult allocation decisions. But we can strive toward a clearer definition of health care. And we can move toward some better understanding of the ways basic distribution principles—*equality*, *equity*, and *need*—govern health care allocation decisions.

Health care: what kind of social good?

To understand fully the distributive justice issues in health care, we first, perhaps, must reach a firmer defintion of *health care*. What is it? Is it a commodity governed by market exchanges among economic unequals? Or is it a *special* social good that stands outside the usual economic rules and principles? If health care *is* special, in what ways is it special? And how do we determine which forms of care are more special than others?

Market-oriented analysts tend to view health care as a *commodity*—as a social good that's bought and sold in a free market like other goods that support, nurture, and protect us. These free-market proponents hold 1) that consumers generally make rational (informed) decisions about their use of the health care system and 2) that the supply side of the market generally responds appropriately to consumers' wants and needs. Health care allocation decisions, they say, are best governed by free-market principles—and deviations from market principles (rights-based approaches, for example) may lead to a coercive redistribution of individual and social resources.

Many (if not most) Americans, however, view health care as a *special* social good that stands outside the standard American market economy. These "special good" proponents make a strong argument. Health care, they say, prevents and relieves suffering—and reduces vulnerability. And individuals need good health in order to seize their opportunities and reach their goals. Although needs change over time and vary from individual to individual, we usually strive to maintain or improve our health, and from time to time we absolutely require medical care services. Thus, say "rights" advocates, medical care is more than a private commodity. It's a primary social good that helps us address the most universal and mysterious human experiences of birth and death—and all of life's contingencies. And, consequently, all citizens possess a moral and legal "right" to health care services.

But a right to what? And to how much? And should we even attempt to frame the national health care allocation discussion in terms of "rights" and "free-market" approaches? Perhaps the discussion surrounding allocation issues requires a more sophisticated understanding of justice—and especially a firmer grasp of the *distributive justice principles* that chiefly govern our allocation decisions.

What is distributive justice?

Justice, broadly viewed, represents a central moral standard in social life—a standard we use to judge both individuals and the basic structure of our society. It has been described as akin to a "human hunger or thirst" and "more powerful than any physical hunger, and endlessly resilient." One theorist defined justice as the "consistent and continuous application of the same norms and rules to all members of a social group to which the norms and rules apply."

The eighteenth-century social philosopher David Hume saw the rules of justice rooted in the sense of general advantage individuals gain from developing a system of mutual constraints on the pursuit of self-interest. Free-for-alls, said Hume, are less advantageous than "regimes of mutual self-interest." And John Rawls, who has formulated the most prominent contemporary theory of justice, calls it the "first virtue of social institutions, as truth is to systems of thought." "A theory," he says, "however elegant and economical must be rejected or revised if it is untrue; likewise laws and institutions no matter how efficient and well-arranged must be reformed or abolished if they are unjust."[1]

Distributive justice, a separate branch of the socio-political justice concept, concerns itself with the ways we distribute the goods and services that affect individual and social well-being. The distributive justice concept centers on the *fairness* of the distribution. And our resource allocation decisions rest mainly on our *values* and our notions of *distributive justice*.

We rarely rely solely, however, on a single distributive justice principle when assessing the justice of some allocation. We usually invoke several principles and then reach an overall judgment by balancing each against the others. A brief examination of three basic distributive justice principles—*equality*, *equity*, and *need*—may help us better comprehend the tensions and extraordinary complexities surrounding health care allocation issues.

Equality

The term *equality* holds various meanings, and we frequently apply the equality principle to health care issues in disparate (often curious) ways. In its purest form, the equality principle would divide all health care resources equally among all citizens—an obviously unworkable formula given the wide differences in needs and desires. Thus, we tend to avoid equal *distribution* discussions and to focus instead on equality of *outcome* and equality of *opportunity* formulations

Most medical egalitarians who argue for equality of health *outcomes*, however, understand the difficulty (indeed, the impossibility) of fully reaching such a goal—given all the differences in individuals' lifestyles, heredities, environments, and other health status determinants. Health care deals in probabilities, and medical practitioners can only attempt to reduce variation in health outcomes—they can't guarantee certainty. Yet, the equality of outcome idea remains a worthy ideal and a utopian goal toward which to strive.

Most medical egalitarians today argue for equal *opportunity*—for equal *access* to health care. And the equal access argument at first glance seems to resolve some basic distribution dilemmas. But access for whom? And access to what? And on what basis? Does equal access mean a claim to *all* potential forms of beneficial care? Or does it mean a claim only to an *adequate* ("a decent minimum") level of care? If so, what constitutes an adequate level of care—and who defines it?

Our quest to establish equal health care access runs headlong into our insistence on preserving the freedom to allocate our personal resources as we see fit. And the collision virtually disables us. The economist Lester Thurow describes the dilemma this way: "Being egalitarians, we have to give the treatment to everyone or deny it to everyone; being capitalists, we cannot deny it to those who can afford it. But since resources are limited, we cannot afford to give it to everyone either."[2]

Equality proponents, who view health care as a basic provision and argue that similar needs deserve equal treatment, frequently find themselves in conflict with equity advocates, who tend to view medical care as another market commodity—available for purchase without restriction in our free-market economy. And this conflict stalls many of our attempts to construct a balanced health care allocation system that meets varying wants and needs.

The equal access principle, a popular but rather mysterious ideal, resolves some of the tensions between the pure equality and equity principles. It satisfies the rule "similar treatment for similar cases" and provides equal access to specific services. But it provides little guidance for deciding on the categories of cases to treat or for choosing between services and target-groups. And our attempts to base health care policies on a strict equality principle often prove difficult (if not impossible)—given all the differences in wants and needs. Thus, Aristotle's dictum "treat equals equally" remains a vague concept until we define equal treatment and specify who is equal to whom.

Equity

We often attempt to resolve dilemmas raised by the equality principle by invoking the *equity* principle, which holds that resources should be allocated to community members in proportion to their investments (time, effort, education, talents, money) in the community, 2) according to their productivity or social contribution, and 3) according to their ability to use a social resource effectively.

Health care equity advocates look unfavorably on policies that seek to distribute health care equally. They favor policies based on the ability and willingness to pay for services; and they seek to extend the private market in health care, to increase cost-sharing by patients, and to rely more upon competition in the medical marketplace.

In its purest form, the equity principle would allocate health care resources solely on the basis of an individual's ability or willingness to pay. But even the strongest equity advocates acknowledge that individuals with great needs and limited resources suffer under strict equity-based systems. And many equity proponents have proposed a market approach that *requires* at least a two-tiered system: 1) a basic tier that would guarantee all citizens a decent minimum level of medical services and 2) another tier that would allow individuals to purchase additional nonbasic services they want and need—and can pay for with their discretionary funds. A tiered system would accommodate some version of the equity and equality principles. But critics of this tiered approach argue that such a system would inevitably drain resources from basic services—and would ultimately would raise basic service costs while reducing quality.

Need

The complex issues raised by the *equality* and *equity* principles are answered in part by the *need* distribution principle. And need proponents advance some powerful arguments. We all fall ill, they say, and we're all susceptible to disability and death. That's our destiny. And although we may engage in certain behaviors that invite dysfunction, we don't ask for illnesses and injuries— and we can't predict when they'll occur. Modern medicine, however, provides highly effective treatments. And since health care is central to the task of attaining or restoring a "fair equality of opportunity" (to which all citizens are entitled), a just society should ensure health care for all who need it—regardless of cost or potential benefit.

But what are health care needs—and who defines them? Needs differ greatly, and in our American consumer society we tend to define many of our hopes, wishes, and preferences as "needs." Moreover, we often fail to differentiate between our "perceived" needs and our "real" needs. Is society obligated to provide *all* of an individual's health care "needs" (perceived and real)—or just a decent minimum or adequate level of care? And, again, who decides? For some citizens, medical need (or necessity, as it's often called) includes *everything* that clinical medicine can accomplish, regardless of cost or prospects for success. Others define need more narrowly and include only those interventions that have proven their efficacy (worth) and their cost effectiveness.

Need has been defined as "the means required for the attainment of urgent ends that are widely if not universally desired." The duty to help another in need or in jeopardy (if one can do so without excessive loss or risk to one's self) is one of a group's natural duties. And, in the words of John Rawls, "In each single instance the gain to the person who needs help far outweighs the loss of those required to assist him." We feel a direct duty to help those individuals who depend on us for their development and welfare and a general responsibility to assist those groups and institutions that primarily develop and care for their members or charges—families, health care institutions, public safety organizations, schools, and the like.

But the attempt to satisfy all needs leads to highly unequal distributions of social goods. *Moreover, as the powers of medicine have expanded, the issue of medical necessity (what we need) and the ends of medicine (what we can accomplish) have become intertwined.* Is the application of aggressive therapeutic intervention in the case of the terminally ill "necessary"—and under what circumstances? How much risk must a patient experience before a hospitalization is considered "necessary?" Our struggle to define the difference between true medical need and the merely medically desirable continues—and with no end in sight.

The expanding definition of medical need—and the increasing ability of medicine to meet those needs—is forcing us to weigh the relative benefits and burdens (both to the individual and to society) of treatment courses. When the benefits of a medical intervention far outweigh the burdens, our allocation decisions proceed relatively easily. But when the interventions begin to strain our resources and deplete other social institutions (education, law enforcement), we face difficult questions. Which health care needs should we consider? How should we prioritize needs? And who decides? Our views on these complex issues frequently change as interventions become more medically effective (and more cost effective), or as certain medical resources become more available, or as we change our judgments about how to distribute a medical resource, or as our individual and family medical needs increase over time.

Many mainstream economists offer compelling arguments against need-based distribution concepts. Health care policies that consider only needs and fail to consider costs, they say, represent a "bottomless pit" that could in time exhaust society's resources. Unchecked health expenditures could conceivably starve our other institutions and ultimately (and paradoxically) impair society's overall health status. Moreover, these critics argue, we cannot rely solely on medical experts and scientific medical knowledge to define our health care goals (insofar as we deliberately define them). We must consider society's economic constraints and its other social needs. And we must consider the tradeoffs we're willing to incur in nonmedical areas of national life.

Health care as a right

Each distributive justice principle, standing alone, satisfies the interests and needs of large social groups. But in our diverse American society (with its diverse health care needs), our allocation system requires the simultaneous contributions of each distributive principle. We must gain a better understanding of 1) the interrelatedness and interplay between and among the three principles and 2) the ways in which each checks the excesses of the others. The health care system has attempted over the years to achieve some balance among the equality, equity, and need principles. But in recent years the *need* principle has begun to dominate. We now define many of our previously held health care "wants" as "needs." And much of our national health care discussion now revolves around a basic question: Do American citizens possess sufficient access to the health care they "need?"

Moreover, we've begun to define many health care *needs* as *rights*—and in so doing we've created some fundamental ethical dilemmas that hold the potential for defeating our most strenuous reform efforts. Do Americans possess a fundamental *right* to health care—and, if so, to what kind and how much? Any claim to certain rights requires justification, and any discussion about rights must begin with some definition of the term.

Over the past several decades, we've expanded enormously our ability to achieve favorable medical results. And many analysts and other citizens now argue 1) that medical care is a social good to which individuals have a right and 2) that it ought to be distributed impartially according to some definition of *need*. But the notion that we possess a "right" to health care begs some questions: A right to what—and to how much? And what is the obligation of others to assure those rights?

A right can be viewed in two ways: as a *liberty* right and as a *claim* right. When we pursue our liberty rights (the right, for example, to exercise one's free speech or to acquire property), we ask only that others stay out of the way—that they not interfere. And when we view health care right as a liberty right—when we ask only that others permit us the freedom to exercise the equity principle and to purchase all the health care we *can pay for*—we encounter little or no conflict. We value highly these liberty rights, and they've played a prominent role in American life.

When we insist, however, on a *claim* right, we impose a *duty* and an *obligation* on others to help us obtain that right. And we ask more than the freedom simply to pursue the claim right without interference. We ask that others contribute their resources, and we ask the state or another guarantor to assure the right. A claim right that lacks a guarantor remains a liberty right—or falls into the category of a need, a wish, or a demand.

Liberty rights and claim rights seldom conflict. But a basic tension exists within the claim rights discussion, and its source can be summarized in this question: *To what extent is an individual entitled to make claims on society's resources, and to what extent is society obligated to meet those claims?* This central tension produces much of the acrimony and conflict surrounding our health care allocation decisions. And we've yet to strike a satisfactory balance between our perceived claims to health care and society's obligations to meet those claims.

Moreover, the cost of claim rights far outweighs the cost of liberty rights, and they're far less palatable to the American public. Tax-based social programs usually involve transfer payments from those with more to those with less. And unchecked health care claim rights hold not only the potential for damaging our other nonmedical institutions but also the capacity for creating even more serious rips in our social fabric. In our attempts to distribute health care more fairly, we've yet to find ways for making clear and consistent distinctions between the obligatory and the merely desirable or good. When are we obligated to make health care resources available to others? And when should we view the sharing of resources simply as a good thing to do—and not a requirement?

And so we are left with basic questions that go to the heart of our allocation decisions. When do wants and interests become needs—and when do needs become rights? What claim does a citizen have to a social resource such as health care? And what is the obligation of other citizens to support (that is, pay) for that right? Many of our policy disputes revolve around these central questions, and the future of our health care system will rest heavily on the ways we define the obligatory and the merely desirable.

Some surveys show that up to 80% of Americans now regard health care as a right. But we must continually remind ourselves that every claim right obligates another citizen, and a society overbrimming with rights inevitably turns into a society overburdened with conflicts. When we introduce an agenda as a "right," reasonable discussion and moderate positions tend to decline.

Moreover, when we claim certain rights without assuming commensurate responsibilities, we begin to act unethically and illogically. Mary Ann Glendon puts it well:

Buried deep in our rights dialect is an unexpressed premise that we roam at large in a land of strangers, where we presumptively have no obligations toward others except to avoid the active infliction of harm. Try, for example, to find in the familiar language of our Declaration of Independence or Bill of Rights anything comparable to the statements in the Universal Declaration of Human Rights that 'everyone has duties to the community,' and that everyone's rights and freedoms are subject to limitations 'for the purposes of securing due recognition and respect for the rights and freedoms of others and of meeting the just requirements of morality, public order, and the general welfare in a democratic society.'[3]

Our Founding Fathers developed a set of liberty rights that protect us from governmental oppression and that generally ensure basic freedoms. Over the years, we've held fiercely to those basic liberty rights, and we prize them highly. But in recent decades, we've steadily extended our notion of rights to include large claim rights, and our appetite for these rights seems at times insatiable. Now, however, we're beginning to recognize that no society can long tolerate an amoral, self-centered, unchecked predisposition toward claim rights. Moreover, as Amitaia Etzioni tells us, those most concerned about claim rights (including the right to health care) also carry an obligation to argue strongly for individual and social responsibility—and for the imperatives of the common good.[4]

Our difficulties in defining a health care "right" and making wise allocation decisions are compounded by our tendency to rely on legal tradition for the protection and extension of our "rights." But legal traditions often provide only limited assistance in helping us grapple with social issues and define the common good. A right, once legally established, becomes an absolute and must be assured, regardless of cost or consequences. In the words of Robert Bellah:

In the American legal tradition, rights are those absolute immunities that prevent tyranny by the majority. But the notion of rights has been extended to include positive claims upon others—claims for equal treatment and claims for such fundamental goods as health care, housing, and food. But casting complex moral or social questions in rights language . . . restricts our understanding of them. Rather than debating the kind of cultural unity and diversity Americans want, the kinds of policies that might reincorporate the desperately poor into the social community, or how Americans will understand economic justice in a centralized, rapidly changing economy, we end up with rigid protections of a limited number of social goods that are understood as inviolable individual rights, with no way to attend to broader questions about our common future.[5]

The courts sustain debates about social questions that our political system avoids. They serve as a forum for a deliberative and transformative politics that our society so desperately needs. But, as Bellah notes, the courts are ill-equipped to perform this function. They lack independent fact-gathering ability, and they decide cases on narrow legal traditions. Consequently, they tend to serve as poor forums for formulating general social policy and framing debates about the common good.

Procedural justice

Our health care allocation decisions are further complicated by *procedural justice* issues. These procedural justice issues revolve around the implementation measures we use to carry out the distributive justice principles. We sense injustice 1) when the health care system favors certain individuals (the affluent, for example); 2) when the providers of health services lack ability, qualifications, and integrity; or 3) when the distribution *rules* and *procedures* for distributing health care resources seem unfair.

Individuals often complain more vehemently about the injustices surrounding distribution *procedures* than about the distributive *principles* themselves. We want to know the rules or criteria that have been used to define the distributive principle—and we

49

want to know who has defined it. If, for example, we conclude that health care should be distributed according to *need*, we want to know the criteria for defining need. How should it be measured? How much is enough? Who decides?

Much social psychological research indicates that individuals who are allowed to participate in the decision-making process are more apt to accept decisions and their consequences. Even though many organizational decisions are often made by representative bodies, when individuals perceive that the decision-making procedures have been made legitimately, they tend to support the distribution principles and practices themselves.

Conclusion

Justice principles address various problems in a society, and they frequently clash and conflict. But they're governed by a common concern: the right ordering of interests and powers within a community. In its own unique way, each principle helps check power interests and reconcile differences. Each contributes both to our individual and collective well-being. And each speaks to specific interests and passions within our pluralistic American society.

Can we point to a distributive justice principle that claims a natural priority and that can give us a more "just health care world?" This question cannot be answered with certitude. Sometimes it's more just to distribute health care according to need. Othertimes it's more just to distribute it equally—or according to the equity principle (ability to pay). Circumstances and community values strongly influence the operative distributive principles. But we must understand the limits (and the potentialities) of each distributive principle—and the complexities that surround each. And we must strive to find the balance among competing distributive justice principles that will give us a more just health care world—and perhaps a more just society.

REFERENCES

1. John Rawls, *Distributive Justice: A Social-Psychological Perspective* (New Haven CT: Yale University Press, 1971), 3.
2. Lester Thurow, "Learning to Say No," *New England Journal of Medicine* 311 (24): 1569–72.
3. Mary Ann Glendon, *Rights Talk: The Impoverishment of Political Discourse* (New York: The Free Press, 1991).
4. Amitai Etzioni, *The Spirit of Community: Rights, Responsibilities, and the Communitarian Agenda* (New York: Crown Publishers, 1993).
5. Robert Bellah et al., *The Good Society* (New York: Vintage Books, 1992), 128.

SUGGESTED READINGS

John Rawls, *Distributive Justice: A Social-Psychological Perspective* (New Haven CT: Yale University Press, 1971).

John Rawls, *A Theory of Justice* (Cambridge: Harvard University Press, 1971).

Morton Deutsch, *Distributive Justice: A Social-Psychological Perspective* (New Haven: Yale University Press, 1985).

Norman Daniels, *Just Health Care* (New York: Cambridge University Press, 1985).

E. Shelp, ed., *Justice and Health Care* (Dordrecht: Reidel, 1981).

4

Balancing Individual Needs and the Common Social Good

Our health care system faces fundamental *ethical dilemmas*—philosophical quandaries that limit our ability to formulate politically feasible and culturally acceptable health care policies. Can we, for example, balance our wish for freedom of choice and our need to maintain family health security? Can we continue to raise our health care expectations in the face of finite resources? *And can the medical enterprise find some balance between its traditional allegiance to individual patients and its moral obligation to the broad common social good?*

These kinds of questions perplex us, and they often engender conflicts that thwart health system change. We've increased greatly our ability to meet the diverse medical needs of our society. But in recent years, our experiences at both the clinical and the societal level have outstripped our traditional ethics models. And now we're facing the need for a more encompassing health care ethics that asks us 1) to weigh carefully the benefits and burdens of treatment (both to the patient and to society), 2) to reflect more systematically and continuously on the norms and values that guide medical theory and practice, and 3) to examine carefully the powerful forces that drive health care costs.

Our medical ethical dilemmas defy easy resolution. But when we begin to understand their sources and to address them with courage and wisdom, we may begin to discover more useful lines of inquiry. And we may begin to construct a resolution *process* that rests less on notions of coercion and individual rights—and more on principles of shared values, mutual respect, and collaboration.

What are ethics?

Ethics has been called "the systematic study of value concepts and the disciplined reflection on moral intuitions and moral choices." It's a philosophical discipline that helps us distinguish between good and bad—between right and wrong—and it's a practical discipline that addresses issues of "oughtness." Ethics helps us define standards of conduct and identify the general principles that underlie those standards. And ethical inquiry helps us find more rational answers to human moral dilemmas and more peaceful resolutions to ethical conflicts.

What are medical ethics?

Medical ethics or *bioethics*—a form of applied ethics—has been called the "taken for granted webs of moral values that constitute the character of everyday life-worlds of medical practice." Medical ethics helps medical practitioners (and others) address moral dilemmas that span diverse moral perspectives. When does life begin, for example—and when does it end? In what ways can we think more usefully and creatively about issues such as euthanasia, abortion, embryo research, and organ transplantation—while respecting and preserving our basic social, religious, and cultural values.

Medical ethics confronts problems that lie outside the strict confines of either medicine *or* philosophy—and it focuses strongly on the *interplay* between medical facts and philosophical reasoning. The discipline attempts to find and clarify the conceptual pre-suppositions that underlie fundamental questions:

- How can we consistently understand right conduct in the biomedical and health sciences—and then justify it to others?
- How can we organize our reflections on birth, repro-duction, illness, and death in ways that will help us address moral questions more effectively?
- How can we make more consistent and sensitive moral, ethical, and medical decisions when all the choices seem problematic?

Certain fundamental ethical principles have guided medical practice over the centuries. We believe firmly, for example, in the sanctity of life and the need to preserve it, and we expect health care professionals to respect and support that central belief. We've also held firmly over the years to the principles of *benefi-cence* and *autonomy*. And some understanding of these two prin-ciples may help us begin defining the tensions between rights-based individualism and the requirements of the common good—tensions that go to the heart of some ethical and economic dilemmas.

Autonomy and beneficence

Throughout most of the twentieth century, the *beneficence* princi-ple—the view that physicians and other caregivers must act in the patient's best interest and in accordance with the ends of medi-cine—has dominated medical ethical practice. The beneficence principle, deeply rooted in the Hippocratic tradition, frequently expresses itself in some form of *paternalism*—an act defined by Gerald Dworkin as "the interference with a person's liberty of action justified by reasons referring exclusively to the welfare, good, happiness, needs, interests, or values of the person being coerced."[1] Defenders and practitioners of paternalism—an action taken by one person in the best interests of another person, but without that person's consent—frequently justify their position this way:

- Many patients choose immediate benefits and short-term gains over possible long-term benefits, even though they may understand that the long-term goals offer greater benefits.
- Physicians are trained in medical problem-solving and, therefore, are better equipped to choose the best course of treatment.
- Physicians are likely to take a more objective stance toward patients' conditions than the patients themselves.

Many practitioners (and patients) still hold closely to certain forms of paternalism. But in recent decades, patients have strongly asserted their *autonomy*—their right to make decisions about their medical treatment. That right, grounded in both common law and the constitutional right of privacy, has been affirmed consistently by the courts, presidential commissions, and other bodies. And over the past several decades, the autonomy principle has come to dominate medical decision-making.

The autonomy principle holds that competent patients possess the ultimate right to self-determination in clinical decision-making and that *their* values, interests, beliefs, and wishes should guide those decisions. This respect for the patient's wishes and judgments—the value we attach to the ethical principle of autonomy—is deeply rooted in both British and American culture. The English philosopher John Stuart Mill stated the principle forcefully in his 1859 treatise *On Liberty*:

> The only purpose for which power can be rightfully exercised over any member of a civilized community, against his will, is to prevent harm to others. His own good, either physical or moral,

is not a sufficient warrant. He cannot be rightfully compelled to do so or forbear because it will be better for him to do so, because it will make him happier, because in the opinion of others, to do so would be unwise, or even right. . . . The only part of conduct for any one for which he is amenable to society is that which concerns others. In the part which merely concerns himself his independence is, of right, absolute. Over himself, his own body and mind, the individual is sovereign.[2]

In American society, the autonomy principle—the right to self-determination—rests on a firm legal foundation. In 1914 supreme court justice Cardozo wrote: "Every human being of adult years and of sound mind has a right to determine what shall be done with his body." And in a landmark 1960 case, *Natanson v. Kline*, the Supreme Court said: "A doctor might well believe that an operation or form of treatment is desirable or necessary but the law does not permit him to substitute his own judgment for that of the patient by any form of artifice or deception."

The right to autonomy and self-determination, however, is not without limits. Sometimes the autonomy right collides with *third party interests*—with the interests of the state, for example, or of family members, health care organizations, employers, insurance companies, or publicly-funded programs (Medicare and Medicaid). And patients and practitioners frequently must factor these third-party interests into their treatment decisions.

Moreover, we all live in some relation to individuals and groups outside the family constellation, and these interlocking relationships constitute the human community. The state maintains a strong interest in preserving this community—and in protecting human life. And it may on occasion either 1) restrict an individual's claim to full self-determination (the right to forego treatment, for example, or to end one's life) or 2) demand treatments that will preserve an individual life. In addition, the state fears the kind of unbridled autonomy that might impair medical practitioners' ability to maintain their professional integrity. And the state allows caregivers to withdraw from individual cases when patients' demands violate practitioners' values, ethics, and standards.

For the most part, however, the autonomy principle dominates, and its emergence as a socio-political, legal, and moral concept has influenced profoundly the shape of medical ethics. The center of decision-making has shifted from the physician (and other caregivers) to the patient—or in some cases to the patient's family. And although today's physicians and other practitioners impose certain criteria on autonomous decisions (the ability to understand information, for example), they generally allow patients sufficient time to deliberate and to make choices. And they generally practice a patient-centered beneficence that places the patient's interest first.

Utilitarianism

Over the past few decades, the *autonomy* principle (narrowly defined in terms of autonomy as freedom) and the patient-centered *beneficence* principle (the view that physicians owe primary moral allegiance to individual patients) has operated within certain implicit assumptions that health care is a *right* to be distributed according to *need*. And these three closely-joined principles or views (usually only implicitly understood) have joined together to form the nexus of a powerful, private dyadic patient-physician relationship that has tended to resist medical care limits and third-party intrusions.

In recent years, however, this absolutist view of the physician-patient relationship has been challenged by a *utilitarian* ethic that seeks to provide the greatest good (utility) for the greatest number. These utilitarians (many of them economists) have begun to promote social policies that maximize society's overall well-being. And their focus tends toward a view that society may legitimately accept harm to a few in return for benefit to the many—and that society must accept the idea of tradeoffs. Utilitarians recognize the finite limits of social resources, and they focus on "the net sum of satisfaction"—rather than on fairness to individuals.

Thus, our pluralistic, individualistic society—enthralled by technology, averse to limits, and resistant to government interventions—finds its national health care reform efforts pulled in two directions. On the one hand, we hold tenaciously to a rights-based individualism that is supported, in Robert Blank's words, by "the belief that individuals have the right to unlimited medical care should they choose it; the traditional acceptance of the maximalist approach by the medical community; and the insulation of the individual from feeling the cost of treatment. . . ."[3] On the other hand we sense (and see) finite resource limits and an increasing need to consider the common good.

Are we hopelessly trapped between two seemingly irreconcilable views: 1) medicine's felt moral obligation to provide unlimited care to individual patients and 2) society's ethical imperative to formulate policies that provide the greatest good to the greatest number. Or are these views too simplistic? Can we find a "new medical ethic" that retains medicine's altruistic commitment to individual patients, while recognizing and responding to society's other commitments and its overall common good?

The new medical ethics and the common good

Traditional medical ethics has focused on the *micro* (or individual) level of moral decision-making—often with little regard for the health care system's social responsibilities. We've tended to ignore the conflict between individual medical desires and broad societal needs—and for some understandable reasons. The society-at-large often seems to medical practitioners (and others) like an unfocused mix of conflicting human pursuits—a fragmented amalgam of interests that frustrates our attempts to see it whole and to define and advance a "common good." Physicians and others who make an attempt to measure the benefits of treatment and to exercise reasonable treatment restraints don't find much assurance that their decisions directly contribute to the overall good. Do the resources saved in the treatment of one patient, for example, really benefit that patient at a later date? Or some other patient with a greater need? Or groups of patients with minimal needs?

Many physicians and other health professionals have side-stepped these kinds of questions by simply defining themselves as the patient's advocate and adopting the view that physicians, in the words of Norman Levinsky, "are required to do everything they believe may benefit each patient without regard to costs or other societal considerations."[4] These physicians devote themselves unswervingly to the patient, and they accept Robert Veatch's view that the Hippocratic tradition requires "the physician do what he or she thinks is in the patient's interest, and does not recognize a qualification such as 'unless the costs are great in comparison to the benefits to be gained'" In Veatch's words, "If physicians are asked to refrain from providing marginally useful care for patients in order to serve society, they must abandon their Hippocratic commitment."[5]

Many physicians find refuge in this patient-centered beneficence, and they continue to think largely in terms of individual patient needs and the traditional Hippocratic strictures. Moreover, our third-party payment system obscures the cost of individual medical services and tends to shield caregivers (and patients) from the relation between medical decision making and social justice issues.

But many physicians and other caregivers today find themselves increasingly caught between their obligations to traditional duties and their felt responsibilities to broader organizational, institutional, and societal goals. And many of these health professionals find themselves in a state of *role conflict* that splits their allegiances. This role conflict—this need or felt duty to meet two sets of expectations (the patient's and society's)—has raised fundamental questions. Can physicians and other caregivers meet the wants and needs (real and perceived) of autonomous patients *and* the imperatives of the broad public good—while fulfilling their professional responsibilities. Can physicians meet diverse expectations—while maintaining their professional integrity?

These kinds of questions press in on us. And the answers seem increasingly clear. Today's (and tomorrow's) physician-leaders face a new and special challenge. They must learn to carry out a dual role, maintaining their traditional allegiance to patients' individual needs—while enlarging their commitment to the social good. And they must learn to operate within a framework that simultaneously places a focus on both individual autonomy *and* the common social good. But how can we design a process that will help us make these difficult ethical and allocation decisions? Perhaps we first need to reconsider our view of autonomy.

Autonomy as freedom

As noted earlier, the autonomy principle—the view that the physician generally must accede to the patient's desires—has largely supplanted the traditional paternalistic ethic. And in our attempts to defeat (or at least push back) traditional paternalism, we have tended to define autonomy in terms of *freedom*—both the "internal" freedom of the competent individual to make choices and the "external" freedom to carry out those choices. In the words of Beauchamp and Childress, this view of autonomy represents the "personal rule of the self while remaining free from both the controlling interferences by others and personal limitations, such as inadequate understanding, that prevent meaningful choice."[6]

This autonomy-as-freedom ethic resonates with deep currents in our popular, legal, and political culture. And it reflects an American individualism that values independence, privacy, self-reliance—and the right to reject outside interference. It treats individual choice as the supreme moral warrant, and it has directly affected the patient-physician relationship.

First, the autonomy-as-freedom focus has given patients the right to define their well-being and to determine the ways they wish to promote their self-interest. That ethic in turn has shielded patients from medical cost concerns. To limit treatment choices on economic grounds is, after all, to constrain freedom—and to limit autonomy.

Second, the emphasis on autonomy-as-freedom has also shaped our expectations of physicians. That is, we expect physicians to provide information and to help us decide on courses of treatment. But we also expect them to advocate for us and to protect us from unwanted outside influences that might limit our autonomy. The result? In short, the autonomy-as-freedom emphasis has given us a markedly atomistic, insular arrangement in which patients expect physicians to address fully their concerns—while protecting them from "intruders" (courts, risk managers, government agencies, insurers and other economic agents) who threaten to limit options or influence choices.

But how far can we push the autonomy principle in an age of finite resources? Is *any* attempt to deny *any* medically acceptable intervention (regardless of efficacy or cost) an assault on the autonomy principle? Or do we need to frame our social world in less constrained terms and develop alternative ways of thinking about our moral lives?

The autonomy-as-freedom view, a bedrock principle of the physician-patient relationship, remains a vital bulwark against paternalism and oppression. But to view human autonomy exclusively or even primarily in terms of human freedom is to miss the pivotal moral feature of autonomy—*responsibility*.

Autonomy as responsibility

Competent human beings possess the morally distinctive capacity to contemplate their values—and to make meaningful choices that reflect those values. This ability to assert a special authorship over our decisions and to bear responsibility for our actions makes us agents and doers—not simply passive reactors to events. And it renders us worthy of moral respect and dignity. It also reminds us that freedom is not the central focus of moral autonomy—it is, rather, a prerequisite for *responsible autonomy*.

In the medical world, our preoccupation with freedom has granted large liberties to patients—but few responsibilities. Patients possess not only the right to decide but also the freedom to decide whether to decide—and whether or not even to hear relevant information. ("Don't bother me with the details, Doc—just tell me what to do.")

Moreover, when the autonomy concept ignores moral responsibility, we find it easier to medicalize problematic behavior and to offer a benevolent hand without condemnation. In the words of Daniel Callahan:

> Matters get out of hand when all physical, mental, and communal disorders are put under the heading of 'sickness' and all sufferers (all of us, in the end) placed in the blameless 'sick role.' Not only are the concepts of 'sickness' and 'illness' drained of all content, it also becomes impossible to ascribe any freedom or responsibility to those caught up in the throes of illness. The whole world is sick, and no one is responsible any longer for anything. That is determinism gone mad. . . .[7]

The medicalization of problematic behaviors has tended to relieve certain individuals of personal responsibility for their actions and to shield them from society's reaction to certain deviant and anti-social behaviors.

Autonomy-sans-responsibility, then, leads to an extraordinarily individualistic view—not only of the physician-patient relationship but also of patients and their social selves. Many moral rights and wrongs revolve around the ways we treat each other, and we define ourselves (in part at least) by our place in the community. But the focus on autonomy as freedom—to the neglect of autonomy as responsibility—has tended to isolate the physician-patient relationship from other real-world concerns. *And it has limited our need to see health and healing in its broad social context.*

A thin and inadequate concept of autonomy as freedom has undergirded much modern bioethical thinking. But we can no longer hold to a simple focus on the dyadic relationship between physician and patient. A new emerging medical ethic asks us 1) to acknowledge the presence of myriad players operating in complex systems of roles and relationships and 2) to see the physician-patient interaction imbedded in a social and cultural value context that now demands consideration of the common social good.

The new medical ethic

Traditional medical ethics has directed its main attention over the years to the moral obligation (the deontology) of the medical profession—to codes of conduct that encompass ordinary moral rules, rules of etiquette, and rules of professional conduct. But in the past few decades, new and more complex moral issues—and new participants in an intensified moral debate—have enlarged the medical ethical sphere. And medical ethics now finds itself subsumed under a new category—under a *health care ethic* that addresses moral issues not only within the doctor-patient relationship but also throughout the health care system and the broad society.

Some analysts now urge us to embark on a deeper public conversation about the *human good* and the *good society*—about issues that will add flesh and sinew to theoretical concepts such as beneficence, autonomy, values, justice, and rights. But the increasingly complex health care (and social) environment and the lack of an integrated moral framework has made it difficult to 1) resolve conflicts between individual and societal perspectives (at both a theoretical and a practical level) and 2) to look simultaneously at individual patient treatment decisions and social good issues.

In the face of these seemingly intractable dilemmas—and in view of the dire need to reduce conflict between individual autonomy and the social good—where then do we go? What concepts will give us a framework for respecting the well-being of the individual while recognizing the imperatives of society's common good?

Citizenship and the good society

Aristotle, who grew up in medical circles and may have completed some kind of medical training, held that all citizens possess both a *private* and a *public* role. The private side of citizenship emphasizes individual rights and interests, and it uses political association to protect and extend those rights. The moral, social, and communitarian side of citizenship emphasizes common purposes and shared vulnerabilities. And it relies on a shared set of loyalties and obligations that support the political community's ends—including the critical ends of health and safety.

In contemporary life, the more private and individual sides of citizenship have dominated medical and health care ethics. But it seems increasingly clear that any workable medical care ethic must acknowledge the contributions and critical importance of both the public *and* private sides of citizenship. If we accept the full idea of citizenship—the idea that we are entitled to the rights and protections of the sociopolitical order but that our allegiances must extend beyond our self-interest—then we must increasingly place health care decisions within a social context that is bounded by limited social resources and competing rights. And we must recognize our obligation to rise above (in Hume's words) "our private and particular situation" and reach a common point of view.

Physicians and other caregivers possess civic obligations. And historically medical codes and ethical principles have defined responsibilities that go beyond the physician's allegiance to his or her patient. The Oath of Hippocrates invokes the sanction of divine authorities and pledges fidelity to teachers, colleagues, and students. And the AMA's Code of 1847 begins this way: "As good citizens, it is the duty of physicians to be ever vigilant for the welfare of the community and to bear their part in sustaining its institutions and burdens."

So there's little new in the idea of citizenship as a source of medical obligation. What's new is the critical need for a citizen ethic to play a larger role in contemporary medicine—and to help bring patient autonomy and societal well-being into a more balanced ethical context. In developing a greater citizen ethic, we may begin to temper our every wish for care and our expectation that we can ceaselessly postpone death. We may begin to initiate more effective processes for confronting and ameliorating a basic ethical conflict between individual autonomy and the common social good. And we may begin to develop a more encompassing health care ethic that recognizes the social context of health.

REFERENCES

1. Gerald Dworkin, "Paternalism," *Monist* 56 (1972): 64–84.
2. John Stuart Mill, "On Liberty," in M. Cohen, ed., *The Philosophy of John Stuart Mill* (New York: Modern Library, 1961), 185–319.
3. Robert Blank, *Rationing Medicine* (New York: Columbia University Press, 1988), 6.
4. Norman Levinsky, "The Doctor's Master," *New England Journal of Medicine* 311 (1984): 1573.
5. Robert Veatch, *A Theory of Medical Ethics* (New York: Basic Books, 1981), 19–26.
6. Tom Beauchamp and James Childress, *Principles of Biomedical Ethics* (New York, Oxford University Press, 1983), 68.
7. Daniel Callahan, *Setting Limits* (New York: Simon & Schuster, 1987).

SUGGESTED READINGS

Robert Veatch, *A Theory of Medical Ethics* (New York: Basic Books, 1981).

Tom Beauchamp and James Childress, *Principles of Biomedical Ethics* (New York: Oxford University Press, 1983).

H. Tristram Engelhardt, Jr., *The Foundations of Bioethics* (New York: Oxford University Press, 1986).

Jacques Thieroux, *Ethics: Theory and Practice* (Englewood Cliffs NJ: Prentice Hall, 1995).

Ann Weiss, *Bioethics: Dilemmas in Modern Medicine* (Hillside NJ: Enslow, 1985).

5

Infinite Needs and Finite Resources:
Cost-Containment and
Rights-Based Claims to Health Care

The tensions between our values concepts (*freedom* vs. *security*), our distributive justice principles (*equality* vs. *equity* vs. *need*) and our ethical perspectives (*individualism* vs. *utilitarianism*) all play out in a competitive, entrepreneurially-driven, politicized health care economic environment that seeks (and finds) ways to meet rising medical care expectations. Infinite needs have collided with finite resources, and we're fast outstripping our ability to pay for all the health care we want and need (or think we need).

How bad is it? Health care expenditures strain belief. Over the past few decades, health care costs have increased approximately 11.5% a year—a growth rate that exceeds any other sector of the economy. In 1992 overall costs totaled $838 billion—13 percent of our Gross National Product and over $3,000 per person. That expenditure will jump 12 to 13 percent a year over the next five years—increases that could give us an annual national health bill of over $1.5 trillion. Health care expenses represent the fastest growing major item in the federal budget, and in the business sector they nearly equal after-tax profits.

The system doesn't simply allow prices to rise—it practically demands it. We've intensely politicized the health care change process over the years, and many cost-control efforts have run into some large contradictions. The public seeks secure and affordable care, for example, but resists changes that limit choice. Various interest groups (business, labor, providers, insurers) seek changes that secure their revenues—but that don't affect their core operations. And legislators and policymakers seek reforms that slow spending—but that don't offend important political constituencies.

Cost-containment plans abound. Some argue for cost-cutting market incentives. Others promote plans that would force employers to provide coverage or encourage small businesses to form insurance purchasing groups. One cost-control approach, pioneered by health maintenance organizations, attempts to "manage" medical care in detail. The management includes such practices as 1) restricting patients to a single primary care physician who must approve all specialist referrals, 2) identifying and reducing variations in practice among physicians and other professionals, 3) preapproving elective hospitalizations, and 4) establishing drug formularies. The Jackson Hole plan promotes a system that uses managed competition and public-private sector cooperation to ensure health benefits for all citizens.

Many of these worthy cost-control efforts merit ongoing consideration and investigation. But they also raise some central questions. And perhaps some of the answers lie imbedded in our belief systems and our expectations for medicine.

1) Americans hold fiercely to their individualism, and they value highly the worth, uniqueness, dignity, and sovereignty of individual lives. This "life-at-all-costs" view reflects an admirable appreciation for the sanctity of human life. But it fuels an individualistic "maximalist" philosophy that frequently fails to consider carefully the benefits and burdens of treatment—and

that often draws resources away from broad collective health care programs. We recognize the need to reduce aggregate costs, but we seem unwilling to limit individual care—a contradiction that creates profound economic dilemmas.

2) Moreover, our individualistic cultural ethos has imbued us with a strong sense of individual rights—including an inherent moral right to health care. But a right to what kind of care? And to how much? We seem willing to constrain spending on certain other social goods. But we seem unwilling or unable to define a "decent basic minimum" level of care that society is willing to support. And our rights-based claim to more and better care continues to override cost considerations.

3) We place great faith in scientific medicine's ability to diagnose and treat our illnesses. And we continue to pour resources into the traditional medical model, despite growing evidence that important determinants of health status (lifestyles, for example) lie outside the medical domain. We assume a tight link between interventions and outcomes, and we cling to a seemingly limitless faith in medicine's curative powers—an expectation that creates increasing demands for expensive specialized medical services.

4) Our belief in scientific medicine's healing powers drives both patients and providers to seek certainty (instead of probability) in outcomes—a quest that often leads to diagnostic and therapeutic excesses. We've yet to move from a "mechanistic paradigm" to a "probabilistic paradigm" that recognizes values and feelings, that provides treatment within the context of a patient's life story, and that gives patients and doctors

decision-making tools for making peace with uncertainty. And we continue to search for costly certainties in a medical world that offers mainly probabilities.

5) Our reimbursement system tends to obscure medical costs through the use of third-party payers—through publicly and privately financed insurance plans that distribute risk and minimize costs to individual patients. Ninety percent of all hospital bills and seventy-five percent of all physician services are paid for by third-party payers. And these payment systems tend to shield both providers and consumers from real costs—and to relieve them of responsibility for identifying and implementing cost-containment measures.

These enduring beliefs and practices (and others—lack of integration among services, administrative inefficiencies, defensive medicine, an aging population, an entrepreneurially-driven system—for example) are imbedded in our social and cultural matrix. And their power and pervasiveness shape our complex economic and political health care arrangements in ways that inexorably escalate health care costs.

Health economists and other analysts have identified the primary factors that drive health care costs, and policy makers and legislators have attempted over the years to isolate and address individual cost issues. But many of these admirable efforts have failed to take into account the systemic nature of our health care services and the myriad ways all the cost-escalating factors interrelate and intertwine. Each issue taken alone defies simple solutions. All the issues taken together pose staggering complexities.

Moreover, we've yet to resolve the differences between two broad approaches for packaging a health care system—two general perspectives that rest on fundamentally different premises:

- Is health care primarily a social, community-based enterprise that seeks fairness, security—and that provides a guaranteed, cost-conscious standard of care for all?
- Or is it mainly a private enterprise (although one with special public policy significance) that emphasizes private insurance programs, individual choice, and the efficiencies of an unregulated free market?

Do we allocate health care resources through the same market forces that govern the distribution of other goods and services. Or do we allocate health resources through planning and regulatory agencies that consider cost-benefit analyses and the political implications of each decision?

Analysts who stand wholly inside each of these perspectives offer firm proposals for resolving our economic dilemmas—formulations that usually prove politically and socially infeasible. In addition, our prescriptions for allocating and conserving medical resources rest heavily on the ideological prism (or model) through which we view the health care system. Sister Rosemary Donley, executive vice president, Catholic University of America, sees four basic models:[1]

- a model that promotes primary and preventive health care
- a model that seeks more affordable care
- a model that advocates universal access to health benefits
- a model that promotes both the individual and common good

Let's look briefly at each.

1) *The de-medicalization model* seeks to check our over-reliance on the medical model (the "care and cure"

branch of health care) and to restrain overspecialization, technology, and the quest for diagnostic certitude. De-medicalization advocates call for less intensive and specialized treatment, more primary care, a greater emphasis on preventive services, and a more rigorous assessment of new technologies.

Reformers who fault high-technology medicine also criticize the dominance of acute-care hospitals, and they argue for more convenient and more familiar places to provide well and sickness care—the schools, the workplace, shopping malls, daycare centers, and homes, for example. This school of thought emphasizes health education, responsible choices, healthy lifestyles, early prenatal care, immunizations, healthy diets, good work habits, regular exercise, safe driving, avoidance of alcohol and illicit drugs—and overall individual responsibility for health care decisions.

2) The *cost reform model* seeks to cut and cap health care expenditures and to revise health care insurance programs. Advocates for this model propose Medicaid expansion for the below-poverty or near-poverty groups, state subsidies that encourage individuals and businesses to purchase health insurance, risk pools for the medically uninsured group, more basic (and low-cost) health plans, and state-mandated and employer-sponsored health insurance for the employed uninsured.

But cost-containment strategies inevitably reconfigure the delivery system. And although cost reform measures may hold the potential for promoting ambulatory care and community or home-based care, cost reformers always aim for cost reduction—not delivery system reform. They mainly promote reforms that reduce (or at least don't increase) costs—even when the proposed cost savings raises quality of care questions.

Many cost-reformers favor some form of universal health care insurance coverage. But these advocates show little interest in augmenting the current open-ended, piecework of health care financing. Instead, cost cutters mainly strive to lower costs and to spread them among large and small employers and between and among the federal agencies and state governments. They also seek to reward prudent management and to eliminate cost shifting.

3) The *universal accessibility model* seeks to reorder health care priorities and to simplify the delivery system. Accessibility advocates argue for a better balance between primary and acute-care centers and for an adequately-trained and culturally sensitive group of primary care practitioners. And they argue that financial barriers (especially inadequate insurance coverage) deprive too many individuals of needed and deserved health care. Certain studies link inadequate insurance coverage to underutilization of available health care services, but the "access problem" frequently goes beyond insufficient coverage.

4) The *professional or personal fulfillment model* seeks to restore certain altruistic values within the health care system. The fulfillment advocates argue that the health care crisis is symptomatic of a more fundamental problem—the post-modern loss of a common belief system and the disregard of moral structures that view human nature as the source of moral authority.

Some fulfillment proponents argue that our disenchantment with the health care system grows out of our unrealistic expectations for the medical care enterprise. Daniel Callahan, for example, holds that the health care system cannot guarantee human well-being and that meaningful health care reform must set limits at both the clinical and societal levels.

Still others argue that the health care system's market and commercial orientation has crowded out professional judgement and altruistic motivation— and has corrupted certain health institutions and health professionals. These professional fulfillment advocates promote a search for a core of humanistic values—a framework that transcends specific reform agendas (national insurance coverage, for example) and that grounds the reform debate in basic philosophical concepts intended to promote both the individual and the common good.

Each of these models contain useful perspectives for viewing proposed allocation policies, and policy makers spend considerable time and effort arguing the relative merits of each. But many of these debates—albeit guided by good intentions and altruistic concerns—fail to consider 1) the ways in which each ideology reflects the values and interests of specific groups and 2) the various ways in which our health care system must capture and integrate important elements of all four models.

Thus, cost-containment proposals seem mired in the tension between and among 1) a rights-based individualistic medical ethic that resists care limits, 2) a broad social ethic that strives to enhance the greater common good, 3) competing views about the nature of health care (social good vs. market commodity), and 4) competing ideological models for viewing the health care system.

Health care and the market economy

We often attempt to apply conventional free-market principles to a health care market that is characterized by non-market relationships. And the health care system frequently finds itself operating in an economic environment that includes neither 1) the *market mechanisms* (cost-conscious consumers, reasonably informed purchasers, etc.) nor 2) the *regulatory mechanisms* (rate-setting, control of supply, etc.) for managing and controlling costs. And we face some large contradictions.

That is, in the non-medical economic sectors, most commercial exchanges consist of two-way, supply and demand transactions between buyers and sellers. Producers and sellers assume a citizenry sufficiently well-informed to make rational choices, to pursue (more or less) enlightened self-interests, and to determine the cost-benefit of a service or product. And through continuous analysis of consumers' choices, the producers supply those goods and services that provide benefits (utility) to the consumers at an acceptable cost—while ensuring profitability (and survivability) to their businesses.

Health care consumers (patients) and health care providers (usually physicians), however, relate to each other in ways that seem to place them outside free-market governing principles. First, patients—often distressed and vulnerable—usually approach the supplier (the physician) bereft of information and dependent on the physician for help in determining their needs (or demands, in economics language). Patients almost always find themselves in need of information—not only about the relation between treatment and health status but also about the *amount* of care (the supply of treatment) and the *kinds* of care that will improve their health status.

Consequently, physicians (operating under the patient's authority and the shield of third-party financing) find themselves performing on both sides of the market: 1) acting as an agent for the patient and supplying information that determines choices (or demand), 2) specifying (or supplying) the forms and degree of treatment, and 3) evaluating the success of the treatment. Autonomous patients frequently help guide the decision-making process, but they're heavily reliant on the physician's knowledge and experience—and they're generally reluctant to explore medical options and other information sources in the medical marketplace. Thus, the physician (not always by choice) heavily influences both the supply and demand sides of the health care market in ways that tend to preclude care limits—and to exclude a utilitarian view that recognizes the imperatives of the common good.

The health care consumer, then, is separated or shielded from the three functions of the usual individual "cost-benefit calculus"—decision-making, cost-bearing, and benefit-receiving. That is, in the health care market 1) the decision-making is highly influenced by the physician, 2) most of the cost-bearing functions are borne by third parties, and 3) even the benefit-receiving is heavily influenced by the physician, who supplies critical information about the goals and expected benefits of treatment.

Potential abuses are held in check by a legal and ethical system that constrains or prohibits certain choices—on both sides. Nonetheless, patients' demands for health care are often influenced by factors unrelated to price and only incidentally related to need. Physicians advise, guide, and persuade as well as serve. Hospitals, health maintenance organizations, and other elements of the "medical-industrial complex" aggressively seek market share through promotions and other strategies. Pharmaceutical manufacturers mount powerful advertising campaigns. And on it goes. Patients become "principals" with many "agents" and a daunting "principal-agent" problem. And many health care demands today are generated by forces that lie outside immediate medical needs and the traditional doctor-patient relationship.

We can and must find ways to economize, but proposed economies often find themselves caught not only between competing values, justice, and ethics principles but also between 1) an individualistic ethic that strives to preserve the traditional doctor-patient relationship and enhance individual care and 2) a utilitarian perspective that seeks the greatest good for the greatest number. And we've reached an ethical and economic dilemma that can be framed with a central question: *How can we maintain patient autonomy and professional integrity while formulating cost-containment policies that inevitably limit certain forms of care?*

The question no longer lies in the theoretical or hypothetical realm. Important and powerful segments of our corporatized health care system have crowded in on the powerful dyadic (near-sacred) doctor-patient relationship that historically has insulated itself from many cost concerns. The health economists and corporate managers play their tune on the aggregate level. But physicians and patients resist the invitation (demand) to impose statistical probabilities on individual cases. And the quiet crisis quietly deepens.

So, what are we to do? How can we resolve basic tensions among competing philosophical principles, conflicting ideological models, and clashing health care and non-health care market place characteristics in ways that will help us restrain health expenditures? And should we even try? The choice seems clear. We must continue to try, and the stakes are high. Peter Drucker, a thoughtful and measured scholar, has noted that the outcome of the health care debate "will determine the very fabric of society and the quality of life in every industrialized nation."

Setting limits

Some analysts, including Daniel Callahan, have proposed policies that would limit care, and their arguments merit some consideration. Callahan poses two basic questions. What kind of medicine is best for a good society? And what kind of society is best for a good medicine?

He answers the first question by noting that good medicine 1) helps assure the viability of a society's social, cultural, and political institutions and 2) attempts to guarantee its citizens a decent baseline of public health and individual care—but beyond that only as much individual care as the society needs.

He answers the second question by observing that health care constitutes only one need among many in a society—and that, by itself, health constitutes no more than a means to other ends. In order to define and fulfill other broad societal needs, a good society, says Callahan, must at some point resist the human desire to overcome all illness and to forestall death through unlimited treatments.

Americans tend to resist imposed limits—in health care and in other areas of social life. Nonetheless, we limit (or ration) health care in a variety of explicit and implicit ways.

We ration explicitly:

- *By age*—when we determine that standard treatments will provide no obvious benefit in terms of improved function or longevity.
- *By prognosis*—when we determine that the burdens will outweigh the benefits of care and when others stand to benefit more from the care.
- *By coverage*—when we treat only those conditions or provide only those services covered by an insurance plan.
- *By scarcity*—When we ration scarce goods (donor organs, for example) and specialized services or construct geographical, financial, and other barriers to care.

We ration implicitly:

- *By budget*—when we limit payment for certain types and lengths of services through capitation and other cost-containment measures.
- *By price*—when we underinsure or when the cost of

goods and services outstrips individuals' or the public's ability to pay.
· *By queue*—when we require individuals to wait for
certain scarce goods and services.

Thus, no longer can we ask *whether* we should limit care—
rationing is here, although it's mainly conducted in implicit and
poorly-understood ways. And as escalating costs continue to tear
at the veil surrounding our rationing processes, we're beginning
to discuss difficult care limit issues—even though strong voices
continue to resist the notion of limits and the development of criteria for limiting certain forms of care.

A two-tier system?

Some analysts and policy makers argue for a two-tier system: 1) a
tier that guarantees an "adequate" or "basic decent minimum"
level of care for all (and that addresses the equality principle) and
2) a set of additional goods and services that individuals can
choose to purchase with discretionary funds (which addresses the
equity principle).

But what constitutes "adequate" and who will define it? And
who ultimately will guarantee an adequate level of medical care?
Tom Beauchamp and James Childress describe the difficulties
this way:

> Despite its attractions, the proposal of a decent minimum has
> proved difficult to explicate and to implement. It raises problems
> of whether society can fairly, consistently, and unambiguously
> structure a public policy that recognizes a right to care for pri-
> mary needs without creating a right to exotic and expensive
> forms of treatment, such as liver transplants. More important,
> the model is purely programmatic unless one is able to define
> what 'decent minimum' means in concrete operational terms.
> This task is, we believe, the major problem confronting health
> policy in the United States today.[2]

Americans have reached agreement that all citizens possess a right to a basic (K through 12) education and that some citizens with special needs (learning disabilities, for example) deserve additional services. Vigorous debates continue over how much we should spend—and on whom. And allocations to the public education system have varied over the years as resources have waxed and waned and definitions of need have shifted back and forth. Nonetheless, we continue to view education as a right—even as we continue to debate the levels we should guarantee.

Health care allocations, however, seem to pose special perplexities. We hold tenaciously to an unstated (perhaps fading) view that health care is a right—and that we're morally entitled to *all* available care. And we tend to reject explicit limits—and any free-ranging discussion about limits. Consequently, we lack a process for concretely defining an adequate level of care and for prioritizing the distribution of finite health care resources. But, a skeptic might ask, "So what? If Americans choose to spend a major portion of their national resources on health care, who's to stop them? Why should we care?" Perhaps the concept of "opportunity costs" may illuminate our need to constrain health care expenditures.

Health care and opportunity costs

Medical decisions are finally economic in nature—a cost-benefit calculation. But our focus on strictly "economic" and "medical" issues may cloud our ability to see health care in its social context and to understand the true nature of health care costs.

In 1795 the French philosopher Condorcet affirmed a view of progress that continues to animate modern scientific medicine. He said:

> Would it be absurd then to suppose that this perfection of the human species might be capable of indefinite progress; that the day will come when death will be due only to extraordinary acci-

82

dents or to the decay of the vital forces, and that ultimately, the average span between birth and decay will have no assignable value? Certainly man will not become immortal, but will not the interval between the first breath that he draws and the time when in the natural course of event, without disease or accident, he expires, increase indefinitely?[3]

We still strive in many ways toward Condorcet's ideal. But we've learned that scientific medical advance doesn't always represent "progress" and may not improve the human condition. And we're learning about *opportunity costs*—about the economic reality that the true cost of a medical service includes the other goods and services that *could* have been produced—but were not.

High health care costs—whether they're 15 percent, or 20 percent, or even 25 percent of GNP—are not in themselves inherently bad. The costs become problematic only when they begin to deplete the other social institutions (education, public safety) that support our overall health status and maintain our social well-being.

Although this pedantic (but important) point may seem obvious, it has policy implications that are less obvious. True cost-containment measures will depend greatly on our ability to see more clearly the social context of health and the ways unchecked "medical model" expenditures hold the potential for ultimately weakening our social environment—and (paradoxically) reducing our overall individual and collective health status. In the words of Leonard Duhl:

> The process of healing involves not only the individual, but the community, tribe, and family as part of the larger social and physical environment. Although we have a responsibility for optimizing the development of individuals toward attaining their health, we have an equal one to look at the healthy development of the environment. To do so requires all our being, from science to art, from the rational to the ambiguous and emotional. Health tests our limits as human beings.[4]

We can't resolve all our economic dilemmas at once—or through the imposition of sweeping public policies. Our complex health care system resists broad change at the macro level. We can, however, begin to establish a process of inquiry (or probing) that will move us beyond "technical" solutions and ideological rigidities—and toward new "mental models" that will give us fresh perspectives and renewed energies. Against the backdrop of value, justice, ethics, and economic principles, we can begin to institute processes of continuous quality improvement at the organizational level that will point the way toward true economies and ongoing change.

REFERENCES

1. Rosemary Donley, "Ethics in the Age of Health Care Reform," *Nursing Economics* 11 (January-February, 1993): 1924.
2. Tom Beauchamp and James Childress, *Principles of Biomedical Ethics* (New York, Oxford University Press, 1983), 279–80.
3. J.M. Condorcet, *A Sketch for the Historical Picture of the Progress of the Human Mind* (London: Weidenfeld and Nicholson, 1955).
4. Leonard Duhl, *Health Planning and Social Change* (New York: Human Sciences Press Inc., 1986).

SUGGESTED READINGS

Sherman Folland, Allen Goodman, and Miron Stano, *The Economics of Health and Health Care* (New York: Macmillan, 1993).
William Kissick, *Medicine's Dilemmas: Infinite Needs Versus Finite Resources* (New Haven: Yale University Press, 1994).
Michael Ignatieff, *The Needs of Strangers* (New York: Viking Press, 1985).
Victor Fuchs, *The Health Economy* (Cambridge: Harvard University Press, 1986).
Robert Blank, *Rationing Medicine* (New York: Columbia University Press, 1988).

6

Meeting Quality Expectations:
The Challenge to Health Care Organizations

The problematic moral, ethical, and economic dilemmas surrounding the health care enterprise remind us again of the myriad ways our health care system lies imbedded in a complex socio-cultural environment. The dilemmas surrounding contemporary health care issues defy simple, formulaic resolutions. And health care policy makers seeking major systemic change face profound philosophical questions that go to the heart of the American value system:

- Can we resolve the competing claims of freedom and security (a value issue)?
- Can we resolve the competing claims of the equality, equity, and need principles (a justice issue)?
- Can we resolve the competing claims of individualism and the common social good (an ethical issue)?
- Can we resolve the competing claims of infinite needs and finite resources (an economic issue)?

Answers to these broad-gauged questions lie imbedded within a cultural, social, institutional, and organizational matrix that powerfully shapes and guides our health care system. And resistance to change can prove fierce at all levels.

At the cultural level, we operate in a relatively invisible "assumptive world"—a milieu in which conventional thoughts and actions appear to constitute a "natural order" that accepts (even guards) the status quo. Although culture possesses dynamic and mutable qualities, changes in our cultural beliefs about health and illness (and resultant changes in the health care system) come slowly—when they come at all.

At the social (or societal) level, we can more readily identify certain factors that directly influence overall health status (education, sanitation, public safety, for example). And we can discern more clearly the social pathologies that burden our health care system. But interventions in the physical and social environments require large, long-term investments that offer few immediate health payoffs. And social policy change (like cultural value change) also comes slowly—and often depends on the ability to achieve broad agreement in a pluralistic American society that resists consensus and social change.

When we turn our attention to the institutional (that is, the health care *system* level), we again encounter staggering complexity. The American health care system—with its broad array of medical service delivery systems and competing political associations of providers, consumers, producers—contains powerful interest groups that work powerfully to block change efforts. Moreover, the rise of medical industry entrepreneurship has given us a "corporate ethos" that frequently thwarts change and innovation. In the words of Paul Starr:

> [this ethos now] permeates voluntary hospitals, government agencies, and academic thought as well as profit-making medical care organizations. Those who talked about 'health care planning' in the 1970s now talk about 'health care marketing.' Everywhere one sees the growth of marketing mentality in health care. . . . The organizational culture of medicine used to be domi-

nated by the ideals of professionalism and voluntarism, which softened the underlying acquisitive activity. The restraint exercised by those ideals now grows weaker. The 'health center' of one era is the 'profit center' of the next.[1]

The complex and stubborn cultural, social, and institutional resistance to systemic health care change often frustrates (sometimes defeats) the most skilled and dedicated reformers. In the face of such intractable (seemingly insurmountable) obstruction and complexity, where then do we go? Where do we begin instituting the incremental changes that eventually add up to meaningful reform? And can we realistically expect to effect lasting change at *any* level of our health care system?

The answer to these questions we think is "yes." We must continue to develop broad social policies that improve education, enhance socioeconomic standing, and promote healthy environments. But, in our view, many of the achievable changes will occur initially at the organizational level and across the continuum of care. And throughout the rest of the book we will focus on ways health care leaders, managers, and other employees can change organizational cultures and continuously improve both quality *and* efficiency. First, however, let's look briefly at the nature of organizations and the special nature of health care organizational life.

What is an organization?

Organizations dominate modern life. Their presence affects— some would say infects—virtually every sector of contemporary social life. The organizational theorist Peter Drucker observes that "Young people today will have to learn organizations the way their forefathers learned farming." But what is an organization?

An organization can be viewed as a system of roles and a stream of activities designed to create a product or service. And these roles—the set of behaviors a person in an organizational position feels *obligated* to perform and that other organizational members *expect* him or her to perform—comprise the structure of an organization. The basic building block is the role, and the pattern of interrelationships among roles makes an organization a system rather than a random collection of roles. A role combines the cumulative formal, informal, technical, and personal expectations about a job. And successful organizations know how to define and coordinate roles—and then move organizational members toward a common goal.

Roles, however, do not provide us with set, rigid scripts. The fluid nature of work and the changing stream of activities in daily organizational life continually require organizational members to modify their behavior and redefine their roles. But when we view an organization as a system of roles (with related functions in various domains and related tasks within those functions), we begin to see more clearly the opportunities for analyzing and revising organizational life—and for effecting change.

Modern organizations find themselves operating in a *Knowledge Society* (to use Peter Drucker's term). Knowledge, says Drucker, has superseded capital, natural resources, and labor as the basic economic resource. And the function of today's organizations is to integrate and synthesize knowledges—and then make them productive. Productive organizations in our modern Knowledge Society create value through *productivity* and *innovation*. They know how to transform knowledge into productive activities—and that is their primary function.[2]

Successful organizations also know (or soon must learn) how to *plan for change*. Our health care organizations find themselves struggling to define their missions in an increasingly complex and often chaotic health care environment. Much of their success—in many cases their very survival—will depend on their ability to build into their structures the *management of change*.

They must learn to examine every process, product, procedure, and policy and ask: "If we did not do this already, would we go into it now, knowing what we now know?" And if the answer is "no," the organization must ask: "And what do we do now?"

The organization must *do something*—not just make another study. It must stay organized for change. And it must build into its social fabric three systematic practices: 1) the ability to *continually improve* its processes, 2) the ability to *exploit* and *develop* new applications from its own successes, and 3) the ability to systematically *innovate*.

Many health care managers and leaders readily accept this broad advice and eagerly seek ways to implement change strategies. But when their high motivations and carefully-formulated plans encounter the daily realities of organizational life, change efforts flounder and hopes fade—and outdated organizational models maintain their tenacious hold. Why? Perhaps the answer lies partly in the special nature of health care organizations.

Health care organizations: some special problems

Today's health care organizations conduct their activities within a dense web of shifting political and economic forces, and they possess special characteristics that confound usual planning and change efforts.

1) Medical providers, inherently conservative, look for strong evidence that proposed structural and programmatic changes will work ("first do no harm"). And they quickly reject potential risk, especially when an adverse outcome might invite legal action. Most change activities, however, usually involve some risk- taking, and successful organizations find a way to move ahead—even when they lack complete clinical and empirical evidence that changes will improve outcomes.

2) Many health care organizations are occupationally structured—rather than administratively structured. From 100 to 200 different professional, technical, or

vocational specialties deliver services. And most are licensed, certified, registered, and in other ways regulated and authorized. This mandatory licensing system rigidly categorizes organizational members and sometimes limits the organization's ability to coordinate and manage services. Moreover, federal and state statutes and various regulatory bodies carefully define the division of labor among occupational groups and delineate the procedures each must follow—a phenomenon that helps maintain a rigid, mechanical, and authoritarian organizational culture.

3) Health care organizations operate under highly complex and fragmented federal and state funding and regulatory mechanisms. Piecemeal and uncoordinated regulations force medical organizations to develop complex internal structures for coping with requirements—an organizational reality that limits the ability to explore and develop innovative care approaches.

4) The reimbursement, legal, and regulatory systems demand meticulous documentation of care—a function that satisfies certain billing and legal requirements and promotes the coordination of care among various providers. But inordinate demands for documentation often reduce organizational flexibility and creativity—and frequently slow innovation and change.

5) Two major "structural interests" now operate in the health care arena: 1) the "professional monopolists" (the medical practitioners and allied health professionals) and 2) a developing coalition of "corporate rationalizers" (health care administrators, planners, educators, and analysts). The professional occupations and associations still dominate the health care scene, but these entrenched interests are being chal-

lenged by a coalition of interests dedicated to rationalizing the delivery of health care services. The conflict—or potential for conflict—between these two groups sometimes inhibits the formulation and implementation of change measures.

We expect our medical and other health care organizations to manage complex problems and to operate in a demanding and dynamic social environment. And many medical care organizations have adapted well to society's unceasing demands. But much of this adaptation has occurred in a rich resource environment—a world that is fast disappearing.

We now must find greater efficiencies and new forms of coordination at the delivery level—within the medical organization and along the community's continuum of care. But what kinds of efficiencies and what measures of quality should we pursue? And can we balance (or at least reduce) the tensions between our quest for efficiency and our desire for quality care? To approach this question, perhaps we first need to define (or attempt to define) *quality*—an elusive concept.

Quality of care: toward a definition

Observers since Plato have struggled to define quality—and still we search. Quality has been described as *innate excellence*, as a phenomenon that *lies in the eye of the beholder*, as *conformance to standards*, and as *affordable excellence*. But these abstract concepts offer little help to consumers, providers, and regulators searching for agreement on the nature of quality health care.

If we define quality as *conformance to requirements*, then the key becomes the specification of the requirements. But who sets the requirements and standards—and how do they decide? If we define quality as a phenomenon that exists in the *eye of the beholder*, then it becomes a highly individualized concept. But whose eyes should we trust? Moreover, the definition of quality changes as values, goals, knowledge, skills, needs, and available resources change over time.

Robert Pirzig in his book *Zen and the Art of Motorcycle Maintenance* sums up some of the confusion about quality this way:

> Quality . . . you know what it is, yet you don't know what it is. But that's self-contradictory. But some things are better than others, that is, they have more quality. But when you try to say what the quality is, apart from the things that have it, it all goes poof! There's nothing to talk about. But if you can't say what quality is, how do you know that it even exists? If no one knows what it is, then for all practical purposes it doesn't exist at all.[3]

Can quality health care be defined? Avedis Donabedian, who has been called the *dean of quality assessment*, recalls a time when this question could not have been asked. "The quality of care," he says, "was something of a mystery: real, capable of being perceived and appreciated, but not subject to measurement. The very attempt to define and measure quality seemed, then, to denature and belittle it." We've improved our ability to define quality, says Donabedian, and there are some elements in the quality of care that are easy to define and measure. But there are also profundities that elude us—and they are, he says, the "secret and glory of our art."[4]

Donabedian calls quality care "that kind of care which is expected to maximize an inclusive measure of patient welfare, after one has taken account of the balance of expected gains and losses that attend the process of care in all its parts." And he sees two basic elements in the provision of quality health care: 1) the technical performance (the *science* of medicine) and 2) the management of the interpersonal relationship (the *art* of medicine).

Excellence in technical performance is directly related to 1) the degree of knowledge and judgment the practitioner brings to the task of *formulating* appropriate care strategies and 2) the degree of skill he or she exercises in *implementing* those strategies. We evaluate technical excellence (the ability to achieve all the improvements in health status that science and technology allow) by comparing it to the practices that produce the greatest improvement in health—to the "best in practice." When technical care produces a poor outcome, says Donabedian, we still must judge it acceptable if it followed practices that were *expected* to achieve the best attainable result.

The *art* of medicine, according to Donabedian, rests on the interpersonal exchange between and among the patient, the provider, and the family members—an exchange through which 1) patients and family members provide information and express their care preferences and 2) the providers share information and invite the patients and their family members into an active collaboration.

The interpersonal process serves as a vehicle for implementing health care, and the success of the care depends greatly on effective management of the interpersonal process. The interpersonal process is expected to respect and uphold virtues such as privacy, confidentiality, informed choice, empathy, honesty, tact, integrity, trust, and sensitivity to individual values and beliefs. And much of the *art of medicine* consists of 1) almost intuitive adaptations to individual needs in technical care and 2) close attention to effective management of the interpersonal process. But since the management of the interpersonal process involves so many different health care providers—who must adapt to so many variations in individual preferences, perceptions, and expectations—specific guidelines don't always serve patients and providers well.[5]

Donabedian finally observes that "quality is a property that medical care can have in varying degrees," but he admits that he's not certain if "quality is a single attribute, a class of functionally related attributes, or a heterogeneous assortment." He also states that "the degree of quality is the extent to which the care provided is expected to achieve the most favorable balance of risks and benefits." When we add cost to this balance, he says, we arrive at a unifying model of quality care: *benefits minus risks and costs.* But, he acknowledges "the identity of the attribute or attributes that constitute quality is not clear at all."[6]

Donabedian's admirable attempts to define health care quality illustrate its maddeningly elusive character. But Donabedian (and other analysts), however, have tended to focus only on the purely *clinical dimensions* of health care quality—on care elements that can be measured by medical outcome. In today's health care organization, however, the quality of health care now also depends on the willingness and ability of *all* the professionals (medical and nonmedical) to improve continually the *processes* and *systems* of care—both within individual organizations and across the care continuum. And our approach to health care quality is undergoing dramatic transformation.

Toward a new approach to quality

Quality programs historically have been driven by the *quality assurance* concept, an approach to quality improvement that Donald Berwick calls the Theory of Bad Apples.[11] Bad Apple proponents believe in "quality through inspection." They rely on compliance audits, motivation programs, and managed care standards; they focus on observed outcomes and non-conforming "outliers;" they attempt to develop inspection tools that will identify malefactors; and they deliver a basic message to employees: "Prove that you are acceptable." Frightened, angry, and sullen workers have played the "bad apple" game over the years. But their defensive response to increasing inspection and discipline has slowed our health quality improvement efforts.

We're now learning that quality problems derive not from the venality and incompetence of workers but from deficiencies in the system and the work processes. Sanctions don't change intentions—and, consequently, they don't improve quality. Rewards and discipline usually fail to improve job design, enhance leadership, or define a clear purpose and vision. And our persistent attempts to sort out the "good" from the "bad" and then assign "blame" has led to disaffection and loss. Attempts to improve quality through inspection have proved at best inefficient and at worst a formula for disaster. And for some good reasons.

First, traditional medical quality assurance efforts have emphasized a conformance to standards approach—an approach to quality improvement that implicitly assumes some acceptable rate of poor outcomes. Standards, however, can prove treacherous. Low quality assurance standards can breed complacency and poor quality; overly high standards can alienate and frustrate providers.

Second, the traditional approach has tended to emphasize physicians' technical expertise and interpersonal relations skills—and to slight the ways physicians contribute to quality through their leadership and their ability to mobilize the health care system's resources.

Third, the quality assurance approach has tended to ignore the most powerful quality tool available: *the ability and willingness of all organizational members to continually and continuously improve processes and systems—within the organization and across the continuum of care.*

In recent years, the quality assurance approach (the Theory of Bad Apples) has lost ground to the Theory of Continuous Improvement—a concept that industrial quality science experts call *total quality management* (TQM). This participatory approach to quality improvement—initially developed in industrial settings—represents a fundamental shift in organizational thinking and quality improvement approaches. And it holds great potential for ameliorating tensions between the quest for quality and the need for efficiency.

In the chapters that follow, we will summarize some of the organizational transformational strategies that quality experts such as W. Edwards Deming, Peter Drucker, Peter Senge, and others have advanced. These analysts and theorists have gained distinction for their work with manufacturing organizations, but their quality concepts and strategies can be directly applied to health care organizational life. And many of their formulations are generating profound shifts in the ways we think about health care quality and efficiency measures.

REFERENCES

1. Paul Starr, *The Social Transformation of American Medicine* (New York: Basic Books, 1982).
2. Peter Drucker, *Post-Capitalist Society* (New York: HarperCollins, 1993).
3. Robert Pirzig, *Zen and the Art of Motorcycle Maintenance* (New York: William Morrow, 1974), 33.
4. Avedis Donabedian, "The Quality of Care: How Can It Be Assessed?" *Journal of the American Medical Association* 260 (1988): 1743.
5. Ibid., 1744.
6. Avedis Donabedian, *The Definition of Quality and Approaches to Its Assessment* (Ann Arbor MI: Health Administration Press, 1980), 327.

SUGGESTED READINGS

Avedis Donabedian, *The Definition of Quality and Approaches to Its Assessment* (Ann Arbor MI: Health Administration Press, 1980).
Marshall Sashkin and Kenneth Kiser, *Putting Total Quality Management to Work* (San Francisco: Berret-Koehler, 1993).
Warren Schmidt and Jerome Finnigan, *TQManager: A Practical Guide for Managing in a Total Quality Organization* (Jossey-Bass, 1993).
A.F. Al-Assaf and June Schmele, ed., *The Textboook of Total Quality in Health Care* (Delray Beach FL: St. Lucie Press, 1993).
Curtis McLaughlin and Arnold Kaluzny, *Continuous Quality Improvement in Health Care: Theory, Implementation, and Applications* (Gaithersburg MD: Aspen Publishers, 1994).

7

W. Edwards Deming and the
Total Quality Management Philosophy

The quest for quality and efficiency—and the need to address simultaneously the requirements of each—has prompted some health care organizations to begin moving from a mechanistic model of organizational life to a more organic mode. The dynamics and goals of these two models (or paradigms) differ significantly:

Mechanistic model		Organic model
1) *equilibrium* (constancy the natural order)	*versus*	*far-from-equilibrium* (tension and) disequilibrium the natural order)
2) *linearity* (cause and effect easily distinguishable)	*versus*	*non-linearity* (cause and effect variant and dynamic over time)
3) *determinism* (information and knowledge leads to certainty and truth)	*versus*	*relativism* (certainty elusive— since observations make observer part of the observed system)

4) *reductionism*   *versus*   *holism*
(system best understood   (greatest knowledge
by examining tiniest   about a system exists
parts and then determin-   not at the detail level
ing how parts fit together)   but at a higher level)

5) *natural order*   *versus*   *constructed meaning*
(there is a natural   (there is no natural
meaning—a single,   meaning—all meaning
grand truth that can   is constructed on the
be discerned)   basis of perception)

The distinctions between the mechanistic (or Newtonian) and organic (or complexity) paradigms—stated here in their most basic terms—represent two increasingly divergent views. And the tensions between the two paradigms hold the potential for stifling change and innovation at all levels of our experience—cultural, social, institutional, and organizational.

The health care system's approaches to quality and efficiency are still rooted mainly in a mechanistic model that holds strongly to equilibrium, linearity, determinism, reductionism, and natural meaning principles. And the system's movement toward an organic model—and a consequent continuous quality improvement philosophy—has thus far proceeded slowly (when it has proceeded at all).

At the organizational level, the Bad Apple Theory (the quality assurance concept) continues to dominate health care quality and efficiency issues, despite growing evidence that "quality by inspection" and "prove that you are acceptable" approaches offer limited payoffs at best—and formulas for failure at worst.

In recent years, the *total quality management (TQM) approach*—rooted in an organic paradigm and the management philosophy of W. Edwards Deming—has gained increasing prominence in health care circles. And its potential for showing the way to systemic health care change and creative innovation merits our closest attention.

Why Total Quality Management?

The *total quality management* concept (TQM) rests on a central and demonstrated truth: customers (including patients, family members, and consumer advocates) seek quality, and successful organizations continuously seek (and find) ways to provide increasingly superior products and services within acceptable cost constraints.

This TQM concept—both a management *philosophy* and a management *method*—rests on three fundamental but sophisticated premises:

1) *Tools*—we can use basic statistical tools, training methods, and behavioral techniques to analyze and improve work processes and systems and to improve continuously the organization's products and services.

2) *Customers*—we must see organizations as complex systems of customers and suppliers (both within and outside the organization), and we must actively and continuously seek ways to identify and understand the customers' needs, wants, and expectations.

3) *Culture*—we must promote the values and vision that foster a humane work environment and the greatest degree of individual and organizational well-being and productivity.

When TQM tools join with a pervasive TQM philosophy, a TQM culture begins to take root—and continuous quality improvement activities begin to reach into all areas of organizational life. Organizational members at all levels begin to analyze and revise production and service processes on the basis of data about the processes themselves. And organizations begin the difficult but interesting journey from a traditional quality assurance approach toward a continuing TQM ethos. But what's the nature of that journey? And what are the specific distinctions between traditional and TQmanaged organizations? Managers and leaders can identify some major differences by posing basic questions:

1) What is the organization's structure?
   traditional = hierarchical and rigid
   TQmanaged = flat and flexible

2) What is the organization's attitude toward change?
   traditional = status quo
   TQmanaged = continual improvement

3) What are the organization's perceptions of supervisors?
   traditional = boss and cop
   TQmanaged = coach and facilitator

4) What are the supervisor-subordinate relationships?
   traditional = dependent
   TQmanaged managed = interdependent

5) What is the focus of employees' efforts?
   traditional = individual
   TQmanaged = team

6) What is the organization's attitude toward labor and training?
   traditional = employees represent a cost
   TQmanaged = employees represent an asset and investment

7) What is the organization's view of quality determiners?
   traditional = managers
   TQmanaged = customers

8) What is the organization's decision-making basis?
   traditional = "gut feeling"
   TQmanaged = facts and data

These questions provide a quick means for identifying the presence or absence of certain TQM elements in an organization. But does TQM really offer managers, leaders, and other organizational members reason for hope and optimism? Or is it simply one more management fad that will soon work its way out of the organizational scene?

We've long searched for management philosophies and methods that might help us create more stable, humane, and logical organizations. In the early years of the Industrial Revolution, "scientific management" promised a more precise, systematic way of increasing efficiency and productivity. The later "human relations" and "democratic leadership" approaches tried to enlist the cooperation of workers. The "management by objectives" philosophy attempted to achieve better understanding between managers and subordinates and greater worker commitment to efficiency and effectiveness. And now it's TQM. But why should we place our faith (perhaps our fortunes) in yet one more management "scheme?" Why should we trust TQM?

The TQM concept has gained great credibility in recent years—and for some good reasons.

First, TQM possesses a proven track record. Surveys and studies consistently show that companies who adopt total quality management practices achieve better employee relations, higher productivity, greater customer satisfaction, increased market share, and improved profitability.

Second, TQM combines and integrates various proven management approaches. American organizations have searched long and hard for more effective management strategies and philosophies. And they have tended to adopt (and then discard) them one at a time. TQM brings together for the first time many of the best management concepts and practices—all of which have proved their worth over the years.

- *Scientific management strategies* showed us ways to measure time, motion, and results.
- *Group dynamics formulations* showed us ways groups can unleash their intellectual and emotional power and direct it toward problem-solving activities.

- *Training and development approaches* showed us ways to develop learning strategies and to design effective learning experiences for adults.
- *Achievement motivation theories* showed us ways individuals and groups gain satisfactions from accomplishments.
- *Employee involvement strategies* showed us ways workers become more responsible when provided the opportunity to influence their work activities.
- *Sociotechnical systems approaches* showed us ways to think of organizations as systems in which each part relates to every other part.
- *Organization development theories and practices* showed us ways to think about change and to help the organization identify and diagnose its problems—and then improve its operations.
- *Corporate culture concepts* showed us ways values and beliefs can influence employees' priorities and work performance.
- *Strategic planning ideas* showed us ways technology can help organizations map their environment and plan their development in a systematic ways.
- *New leadership theories* showed us ways to distinguish between leading and managing—and to mobilize human effort through vision, trust, and empowerment.

Each of these management concepts has demonstrated some worth—and some limitations. The TQM philosophy has borrowed some of the best features of each and included them in its theoretical base (a kind of inclusive mosaic).

Third, TQM is consistent with values we admire. TQM is based on a humanistic value system, and it begins with the mandate that organizations must treat customers, employees, and

vendors fairly—and that all organizational members must understand the need to work cooperatively and move collectively
toward a common vision. TQM, then, represents more than a
management method and set of management tools. It represents a
management philosophy and an *organizational culture* that asks
all employees to transform problems into opportunities—and to
keep improving continuously the organization's processes and
systems.

TQM (both a set of social tools and a management philosophy) represents an organizational cultural paradigm shift—a
fundamental change in organizational values and priorities that
fosters a humane and satisfying work environment and that promotes efficiency and quality. And no one has more to say about
TQM philosophy than W. Edwards Deming.

W. Edwards Deming and the TQM idea

W. Edwards Deming—the driving force behind the TQM concept—
first gained international prominence through his contributions
to the post-World War II Japanese industrial revitalization. In the
early 1980s, American manufacturing and service sectors began
to discover Dr. Deming's approaches to quality improvement.
And in recent years, his quality and efficiency concepts have
reached into important areas of American commercial life—
including the health care industry. We can only briefly summarize
Deming's concepts here, but we hope this introduction to his
powerful philosophy will provide a basis for exploring the TQM
idea—and for relating TQM to the health care service mission.
The concepts and principles described here are taken from his
seminal book *Out of the Crisis*.[1]

For Deming, insightful management rests on an "awareness
process" he calls *profound knowledge*. The process consists of
four interdependent and interactive components: 1) *appreciation*

for a system, 2) *theory of variation*, 3) *theory of knowledge*, and 4) *psychology*. Let's look briefly at each.

Appreciation for a system

Deming views a system as "a network of functions or activities that work together for the aim of the organization." An organization cannot function effectively, he says, without 1) a clear mission communicated clearly to all organizational members and 2) full cooperation among components in the system.

Deming assigns managers the responsibility for optimizing systems through creating an organizational culture that helps all members 1) clarify relationships between system components, 2) define connections between processes, and 3) gain insights into interactions. The systems approach helps managers and other organizational members understand that all work processes contain suppliers (who provide inputs) and customers (who use the outputs). "Internal customers" (other employees) use the outputs of a process *within* the system. "External customers" (the conventional consumers) purchase the ultimate products or services of the system. And the quest to reduce variation among process inputs—people, methods, machines, materials, measurements, and environmental factors—lies at the heart of the TQM idea.

Theory of variation

Variation in a process derives from *common causes and special causes*. And the ability to distinguish between the two is an important key to successful TQM implementation. Deming estimates that only 6% of all problems derive from special causes. Most improvements, he says, will derive from addressing common causes of variation within the processes. Deming insists that managers must possess some means for distinguishing between special and common causes of variation. And he strongly maintains that statistical methods can provide the primary tool for making that distinction. In Deming's words, "Management is prediction!" A process in statistical control is stable, says Deming, and a stable process provides a rational basis for prediction. (We'll say more about special and common cause variation in Chapter 9.)

Psychology

TQM tools and techniques (control charts, for example) help organizational members 1) learn the meaning of variation, 2) understand that output variation derives from numerous process inputs, and 3) identify the presence of special and common causes of variation. And TQM tools contribute to quality in some direct and obvious (and quantifiable) ways. But TQM also provides a critical *psychological* benefit that goes far beyond the benefits associated with a structured approach to quality issues.

TQM increases competence and a sense of control over work outcomes, and it helps employees move from a passive to a proactive stance. This proactive involvement— and resultant sense of control over work processes and work outcomes—creates in turn a sense of *self-confidence* and *self-esteem*. And this sense of *self-efficacy* (together with skill development) promotes enjoyment, personal growth, and true job satisfaction—and it ultimately fosters a more psychologically healthy and humane organizational culture.

Theory of knowledge

Deming's Second Theorem declares, "We are ruined by best efforts misdirected." And Deming insists that theory should guide management activities. In his words, "Theory leads to questions. Without questions, experience and examples teach nothing. Without questions, one can have only an example. Copying an example of success without understanding it with the aid of theory, may lead to disaster." He also claims, "There are no short-cuts to mastery of subject matter; there is no substitute for knowledge." Deming expects managers to address issues that cannot be objectively measured. And he frequently quotes Lloyd S. Nelson, who noted: "The most important figures [statistics] for management are unknown and unknowable."

Profound knowledge then represents a system in itself—a system whose components are interdependent and interactive and whose aim is optimum organizational performance. And Deming's *Fourteen Points for Management* provide a powerful method for developing and implementing profound knowledge in the workplace.

The Fourteen Points of Management

The Fourteen Points represent a code of conduct and a value system that provides a frame of reference for viewing organizational change. The TQM journey toward innovation, says Deming, requires faith in a future. And how else, he asks, can we deal with the invisible and unknowable except through faith? Although Deming's management principles have been applied mainly to the manufacturing sector, service organizations—including health care organizations—can draw insights from his Fourteen Points. Taken together, the points provide a tool for predicting the future and making a commitment to continuous quality improvement.

Point 1: *Create constancy of purpose for improvement of product and service.*

Management faces two sets of problems, Dr. Deming says: those of today and those of tomorrow. "It is easy to stay bound up in the tangled knots of the problems of today, becoming ever more and more efficient in them." Organizations formulate mission statements and long-term strategic plans that express constancy of purpose. But too often, declares Dr. Deming, they stay "on the shelf, dust covered."

To establish constancy of purpose, organizations must 1) innovate, 2) conduct research and education activities, 3) improve continuously their products and services, and 4) invest in equipment and other production and service aids. In Deming's words:

> People are concerned about the future, and the future is ninety days at the most, or nonexistent. There may not be any future. That is what occupies people's minds. That is not the way to stay in business. Not the way to get ahead. You have to spend some time on the future. And to put it off—'Nothing could happen today anyway. Could just as well put it off anther day, another week, no harm done because nothing would happen anyway today.' So you put it off and put it off and nothing happens.

Point 2: *Adopt the new philosophy.*

Dr. Deming suggests that modern corporations must believe in quality the way they once believed in progress—and they must pursue new management philosophies. In his words:

> Point 2 really means in my mind a transformation of management. Structures have been put in place in management that will have to be dismantled. They have not been suitable for two decades. They never were right, but in an expanding market you couldn't lose. The weaknesses showed up when competition came in. We will have to undergo total demolition of American style of management, which unfortunately has spread to just about the whole western world. In fact, one problem is that American companies have forced it on to their Canadian subsidiaries and subsidiaries in other countries, thus injecting disease the world over. This is a pity.
>
> Competition introduced a squeeze, Management offered all kinds of excuses. There was every kind of thing in this world, except the awful truth that Americans were beaten. Where they have been beaten is in the management. It has been focusing on results.

Point 3: *Cease dependence on mass inspection.*

Certain forms of periodic inspection *can* improve quality. But efforts to improve quality through *mass inspection* (especially final product inspection when defects in the process cannot easily be identified) usually prove too late, too ineffective, and too costly. Quality grows out of improvements in processes and reductions in variation. And Deming insists that ever decreasing variation decreases total cost. Two products or services, however, may meet the same specifications but differ so much that one possesses quality and the other does not. Dr. Deming illustrates the point this way:

> Down the road, there's a music store, and that music store would be delighted to sell you the score for a 140-piece orchestra—Beethoven's Fifth Symphony. Listen to the London Symphony Orchestra play it. So wonderful. Now listen to my hometown orchestra play it. Just listen to the difference. The London Symphony . . . the hometown orchestra. Same music; same specifications. Not a mistake. Both perfect. But listen to the difference. Just listen to the difference.

Point 4: *End the practice of awarding business on the basis of price tag alone.*

A price tag, notes Dr. Deming, is unambiguous and therefore appealing. But quality improvement depends on the ability to select superior suppliers and to reduce the potential for variation. The attempt to drive down every purchase price can drive good vendors and services out of business—and ultimately prove costly. John Ruskin, the nineteenth century English critic and author put it this way:

> It's unwise to pay too much, but it's worse to pay too little. When you pay too much, you lose a little money—that's all. When you pay too little, you sometimes lose everything, because the thing you bought was incapable of doing the thing it was bought to do.

Point 5: *Improve constantly and forever the system of production and service.*

The principle of continual improvement lies at the heart of Deming's philosophy. All organizational members (but especially managers), says Deming, must constantly seek ways to improve work processes and systems. But simply meeting specifications and avoiding and eliminating special cause variation will not ultimately improve quality. In Dr. Deming's words:

> Putting out fires is not improvement. Finding a point out of control, finding the special cause and removing it, is only putting the process back to where it was in the first place. It is not improvement of the process. You are in a hotel. You hear someone yell fire. He runs for the fire extinguisher and pulls the alarm to call the fire department. We all get out. Extinguishing the fire does not improve the hotel. That is not improvement of quality. That is putting out fires.

Point 6: *Institute training.*

Training provides managers and other organizational members with the tools they need to evaluate processes and improve systems. Training improves processes and reduces variation—and thus increases quality. But managers must learn that 1) people learn in different ways and that 2) once a process has been brought into statistical control (once its output is predictable) further training *by the same method* will not help workers improve the process. Dr. Deming puts it this way:

> A woman said she couldn't find out what the job was. I said, 'Well, how did you find out?' Her companions helped her. They taught her what was right and what was wrong. How could they teach her anything else but the way that they were doing it, some ways of which were right and some wrong? They didn't know; she couldn't know. It's just like taking lessons on the piano from someone who never had a lesson on the piano. He learned by

himself how to play. If you take lessons from him, you will learn a lot that is wrong; you might learn some that is right. Neither pupil nor teacher will know what is right and what is wrong. Did you know that when this happens, and it is going on all around us, the training gets worse and worse?

Point 7: *Adopt and institute leadership.*

The leadership theorist Warren Bennis notes: "Managers do things right; leaders do the right things." Effective leaders create, embody, and communicate an organization's vision, values, and mission. They clarify the path that organizations and organizational members must follow to achieve their mutual objectives—and to drive systems toward optimization. In Dr. Deming's words:

> People come into a company from college, learn about the company by going in and being supervisors somewhere. Pity poor people that have such supervision. No help at all! Aren't they entitled to some help? Where is the supervisor who knows how to find who is in need of individual attention? Show me one. There is no such thing as supervision, and should not be, unless people know how to supervise.
>
> There is no excuse to offer for putting people on a job that they know not how to do. Most so-called 'goofing off'—somebody seems to be lazy, doesn't seem to care—that person is almost always in the wrong job, or has very poor management.

Point 8: *Drive out fear.*

Deming claims that "no one can put in his or her best performance unless he or she feels secure." Fear begets misinformation, hidden agendas, and padded numbers—and it reduces system optimization. Fear-driven employees often focus on meeting specifications, quotas, guidelines, and regulations at the expense of the organization's best interests. Dr. Deming says:

What are people afraid of? Afraid to contribute to the company. Better not get out of line. Don't violate procedures. Do it exactly this way.

Why don't they complain to manufacturing about stuff that comes in already defective, hard to work with? No matter what you do, you can't turn out quality work—not within the time allowed. Why don't they say something about that?

Look. Complain to the foreman about it, he can do nothing. Totally helpless about it. You only advance yourself on his list toward the top. And if he has to do some cutting, he begins at the top. Gets rid of the nuisance makers. Asking too many questions that he can't answer will only embarrass him. People don't complain. They don't complain. They have jobs.

Fear takes a horrible toll. Fear is all around, robbing people of their pride, hurting them, robbing them of a chance to contribute to the company. It is unbelievable what happens when you unloose fear.

Point 9: *Break down barriers between staff areas.*

Barriers reduce team work and breed suboptimization. They interfere with the ability of all components and processes to recognize their systemic function and to provide feedback about the ways their activities affect system performance. But barriers tend to dissolve when all workers understand customers' needs and expectations and when they see the ways their individual contributions advance the organization's overall goals. Says Dr. Deming:

> Is it management's job to help staff areas work together? To promote teamwork? Sounds great, but it can't be done under the present system. In spite of the system, you will find teamwork. But when it comes to a showdown under the present system and someone has to make a decision—his own rating or the company's—he will decide for himself. Can you blame him? People work in the system. Management creates the system.

Point 10. *Eliminate slogans, exhortations, and targets for the work force.*

Slogans, exhortations, and numerical goals, says Deming, never improve work performance—and, in fact, ultimately offend employees and "generate frustration and resentment." Moreover, these cheerleading gimmicks and arbitrary objectives fail to take into account the influence of processes and systems. In Dr. Deming's words:

> It is totally impossible for anybody or for any group to perform outside a stable system, below or above it. If a system is unstable, anything can happen. Management's job, as we have seen, is to try to stabilize systems. An unstable system is a bad mark against management.
>
> You can beat horses; they run faster for a while. Goals are like hay somebody ties in front of the horse's snout. The horse is smart enough to discover no matter whether he canters or gallops, trots, or walks, or stands still, he can't catch up with the hay. Might as well stand still. Why argue about it? It will not happen except by change of the system. That's management's job, not the people's.

Point 11: *Eliminate numerical quotas.*

Deming call quotas "a fortress against improvement of quality and productivity." And he says, "I have yet to see a quota that includes any trace of a system by which to help anyone do a better job." Quotas fail to consider quality and to provide data that improves the system. And they destroy pride in workmanship. Organizations need goals, aims, and objectives—but they don't need arbitrary numerical goals. Instead of assigning quotas to a job, says Deming, managers should study the work and define the limits of the job—and then work to reduce variation and help employees increase output. In Dr. Deming's words:

Where are the hangups? Study the records. What is taking the time? What is the difference between people who have been there three years versus two years? Maybe you can learn something. There will be a distribution of results. They will not all come up to the average. No matter what, half of them will be below. The problem is to improve the system and find out who is having the trouble.

Isn't it clear? Numerical quotas—so many per day; a plant manager—so many per day. If he fails to meet it, he fails. No regard for what is a day's work. No possibility to improve. Do you think a plant manager will report 7,000 when the quota is 5,000? That he will report 5,500 when the quota is 5,000? No. Put them under the counter. May need them for a rainy day. It may rain tomorrow.

Point 12: *Remove barriers that rob people of pride of workmanship.*

Too many organizations treat employees as commodities and rob them of opportunities to take pride in their work. But workers know that their jobs depend on the quality of their organization's products or services, and they resent managers' indifference to their needs for excellence and quality. Dr. Deming says:

> In a meeting of two hundred factory workers, a man said to me, 'It is a matter of communication.' I said, 'Tell me about it.' His machine had gone out of order and would make only defective items. He had reported it, but the maintenance men could not come for a long time. Meanwhile, he was trying to repair it himself. The foreman came along and said to run it. 'In other words, he told me to make defective items.'
>
> 'Where is my pride of workmanship?' he asked me. 'If the foreman would give me as much respect as he does the machine, I'd be better off.'
>
> He didn't want to get paid for making defective items.
>
> Talk about motivation. People are motivated. All people are motivated. Everyone? No. There are exceptions. Some are beaten down so often, so many times, that they have lost, temporarily at least, interest in the job.

Point 13: *Institute a vigorous program of education and retraining.*

Quality begins and ends with education. Applied knowledge improves systems. And in Deming's words, "In respect to self-improvement, it is wise for anyone to bear in mind that there is no shortage of good people. Shortage exists at the high levels of knowledge; this is true in every field." Committed, knowledge-able people optimize systems. Good managers view them as an asset—not an expense. And they recognize the ongoing need for education and retraining programs that improve professional competencies and the quality of organizational life. Dr. Deming says:

> How do you help people to improve? What do you mean by im-prove? If you ask me, I would say that I find a general fear of edu-cation. People are afraid to take a course. It might not be the right one. My advice is take it. Find the right one later. And how do you know it is the wrong one? Study, learn, improve. Many companies spend a lot for helping their people in this and that way. In arithmetic, geology, geography, learning about gears.
>
> You never know what could be used, what could be needed. He that thinks he has to be practical is not going to be here very long. Who knows what is practical?
>
> Help people to improve. I mean everybody.

Point 14: *Take action to accomplish the transformation.*

Managers must ensure that all organizational members under-stand the Fourteen Points, and then they must take action to ad-vance the points and begin the process of continual improvement. But how does the organization initiate action? Deming rec-ommends the Shewart Cycle—sometimes called the "Plan, Do, Check, Act (PDCA) cycle." The PDCA cycle consists of four steps:

- *Step 1:* Study a process and determine the changes that might improve it? Determine whether tests or data are needed.
- *Step 2:* Carry out the tests or make the change on a small scale.
- *Step 3:* Observe the effects.
- *Step 4:* Determine the results of the test (What did observers learn?). Repeat tests if necessary—perhaps in a different environment. Look for side effects.

The Shewhart Cycle (little more than a straightforward rational problem-solving process) helps identify special causes of variation in a process, and it leads, says Dr. Deming, to "continual improvement of methods and procedures."

Conclusion

The TQM concept embraces and attempts to implement both a set of tools *and* a philosophy of management. TQM tools and techniques—the most visible evidence of the TQM presence—contribute strongly to quality and efficiency programs. But they can't by themselves assure TQM. Nor can a top-down imposed TQM management philosophy by itself ensure quality improvement. But when tools and philosophy combine in creative and effective ways, they begin to foster a TQM *culture*—a set of values that directs the organization's ethos 1) away from the view that managers control work performance through a system of rewards and punishments and 2) toward the view that managers and other organizational members must continually seek to improve processes.

This fundamental shift in values represents the first step in a TQM journey that helps organizations adapt to change, achieve goals, and coordinate employees' work efforts. In his compelling book, *The Fifth Discipline: The Art and Practice of the Learning Organization*, Professor Peter Senge describes five disciplines that can help move organizations toward a true TQM culture. His vision speaks directly to health care quality and efficiency issues—and his insights point the way toward a brave new organizational future.

REFERENCES

1. W. Edwards Deming, *Out of the Crisis* (Cambridge MA: Massachusetts Institute of Technology, 1991).

SUGGESTED READINGS

W. Edwards Deming, *Out of the Crisis* (Cambridge MA: Massachusetts Institute of Technology, 1991).

Rafael Aguayo, *Dr. Deming, the American Who Taught the Japanese About Quality* (New York: Carol Publishing Group, 1990).

Mary Walton, *The Deming Management Method* (New York: Perigree Books, 1986).

Stephen Shortell and Arnold Kaluzny, *Health Care Management: Organization Design and Behavior* (Albany NY: Delmar Publishers, 1994).

William Scherkenbach, *The Deming Route to Quality and Productivity* (Milwaukee: Ceep Press, 1986).

Henry Neave, *The Deming Dimension* (Knoxville TN: SPC Press, 1990).

8

Peter Senge and the Learning Organization

In his book *The Fifth Discipline: The Art & Practice of the Learning Organization*, Peter Senge, Director of the Systems Thinking and Organizational Learning Program at the Massachusetts Institute of Technology's Sloan School of Management, describes the dynamics of the *learning organization*. His insights offer a powerful new approach to organizational work life. And they provide valuable guidance for health care leaders and managers seeking to develop a new form of participative management—and to move toward an organizational culture that fosters creative and continuous change.

Our modern organizations labor, in Senge's view, under *learning disabilities* that prevent them from recognizing threats and seizing opportunities. Good ideas and promising experiments languish and never finally take root. Managers blame their problems on external events and ignore long-standing conditions that have (or soon will) put their organizations into decline. And organizational members hold tenaciously to outdated thinking.

We persistently try, Senge says, to break complex tasks and subjects into manageable pieces—and we frequently lose sight of "the big picture." But when we shed the illusion that the world is composed of separate, unrelated forces, we begin to think systemically and to see coherent wholes. Moreover, we begin to see opportunities for building *learning organizations*—for creating organizational cultures that promote creativity and innovation.

The new innovative, learning organizations, says Senge, are shaped by five separate disciplines or "component technologies" that work together like an ensemble. Senge terms these disciplines *personal mastery, mental models, shared vision, team learning,* and *systems thinking.* And the descriptions of these disciplines are taken from Professor Senge's seminal book *The Fifth Discipline: The Art & Practice of the Learning Organization.*[1]

Personal mastery

Personal mastery—a lifelong discipline of personal growth and learning—goes beyond skill development and spiritual unfolding. Personal mastery fosters a creative (rather than a reactive) approach to life, and when it becomes a discipline—an activity we integrate into our daily lives—it embodies two elements: 1) the ability to clarify continually our vision (what we want) and 2) the ability to see clearly our current reality (where we are relative to what we want). Individuals who acquire personal mastery create the spirit of the learning organization, and they share some basic characteristics:

- They continually clarify and deepen their personal vision.
- They live in a continual learning mode—they never "arrive."
- They stay acutely aware of their ignorance, their incompetence, their growth areas.
- They remain deeply self-confident and committed.
- They take initiative.
- They learn quickly.
- They take risks.

- They delay gratifications.
- They act out of firmly-held values.
- They exhibit a broad and deep sense of responsibility toward their work.
- They focus their energies
- They develop patience.
- They are deeply inquisitive.
- They view reality clearly and embrace it as an ally.
- They embrace innovation and work with forces of change.
- They possess a special sense of purpose that is supported by visions and goals.
- They feel connected to others and to life itself and yet sacrifice none of their uniqueness.
- They feel connected to a larger creative process they can influence but cannot unilaterally control.
- They make commitments to goals larger than themselves.

Organizations that promote personal mastery and employee development establish a covenantal relationship with their members—a bond that goes beyond the traditional contractual relationship ("an honest day's pay for an honest day's work"). The covenantal relationship rests on a shared commitment to ideas, issues, values, goals, and management processes. It promotes unity, grace, and poise—and it seeks to develop fully the organizational members' personal and professional capabilities.

Some organizations discourage personal mastery. They consider the discipline "soft" and grounded in unquantifiable concepts such as intuition and personal vision. Many managers view personal mastery as a threat to the organization's established order—and their fear is often justified. Empowered employees operating in an organization that lacks a common vision may increase organizational stress and incoherence—and certain employees may begin to challenge the established order. Leaders and managers, however, who build a shared vision and promote personal mastery reduce stress and increase organizational alignment, coherence, and direction.

Personal mastery rests on the ability to connect with our ultimate intrinsic desires—not simply with our secondary goals. Indeed, much of our potential for happiness may derive from the ability to live consistently with our purpose. The playwright George Bernard Shaw put the idea this way:

> This is the true joy in life, the being used for a purpose recognized by yourself as a mighty one . . . the being a force of nature instead of a feverish, selfish little clod of ailments and grievances complaining that the world will not devote itself to making you happy.[2]

Personal mastery requires the ability to focus and refocus on one's true desires—on one's purpose and vision. Most of us, however, are acutely (sometimes painfully) aware of the gap between vision and reality. This gap can make a vision seem unrealistic or fanciful, and it can lead to discouragement and despair. But the gap between vision and current reality—a gap we might term *creative tension*—can also serve as a source of creative energy.

The principle of creative tension lies at the center of personal mastery and integrates all elements of the discipline. We can use creative tension—the gap between our personal vision and our personal reality—to generate energy for change. And the mastery of creative tension can produce some big payoffs.

1) It can transform the way we view "failure." When we see failure only as a gap between vision and reality, perceived failure simply represents a shortfall, an opportunity to learn—about inaccurate pictures of current reality, about strategies that didn't work, and about the clarity of our vision. When we view "failure" as an opportunity, we rob it of its power to reduce our worth and strength.

2) It leads to a fundamental shift in our whole posture toward reality and turns current reality into an ally. It reduces distortions in our perceptions of reality and helps us remain true to our vision and our commitment to truth—vital forces in generating creative tension.

3) It brings out a capacity for perseverance and patience, and it makes time an ally.

How can leaders help organizational members develop personal mastery? They can work relentlessly to foster an organizational culture that values education, vision creation, inquiry, commitment to truth, and challenges to the status quo. Such an organizational culture will strengthen personal mastery in two ways: 1) it will continually promote personal growth and 2) it will provide the educational opportunities organizational members need to grow and develop. The core leadership strategy is simple: *be a model.* Commit to one's own personal mastery—to one's own learning opportunities and personal growth.

Mental models

Why do so many good plans, sound strategies, and systemic insights never finally take root? Can we continue to blame our organizational deficiencies on poor management and weak leadership? Or do we need to investigate our *mental models*—the deeply ingrained assumptions, generalizations, and even pictures and images that shape our world view and influence our actions. These mental models often lock us into familiar but outdated and ineffective ways of thinking and acting. And our success in developing learning organizations will depend greatly on our ability to manage mental models—to surface, test, and change our beliefs and assumptions.

Our mental models determine not only how we make sense of

the world but also how we take action. Although people do not always behave congruently with their espoused theories (what they say), they tend to behave congruently with their theories-in-use (their mental models). Mental models, then, are *active*—they shape what we see and, consequently, what we do. But we observe selectively—when we observe at all. And many organizational problems derive from our inability or unwillingness to surface mental models and to examine carefully their nature and influence.

Organizations frequently develop chronic gaps between their mental models and reality. Deeply entrenched models can overwhelm even the best systemic insights—and ultimately undermine change activities. But if mental models can impede learning, can they not also accelerate learning? In recent years, many business corporations have given serious attention to this question. And more than a few have gained competitive advantage through helping managers clarify their assumptions and uncover internal contradictions—and then formulate new strategies based on fresh assumptions and systemic thinking.

The traditional authoritarian organization has emphasized the managing, organizing, and controlling functions. The new learning organization emphasizes a common vision, shared values, leadership, personal mastery—and challenges to established mental models. And this new modern organization, seeking always to help managers and other organizational members reflect *together* on their current mental models, helps all employees 1) bring prevailing assumptions into the open, 2) examine their biases, 3) experiment collaboratively with new ways of thinking, and 4) develop the best possible mental models for any circumstance.

To develop an organization's capacity to work with mental models, effective managers and leaders must institute education programs that develop new skills—and then implement programs of planned change. Effective learning organization leaders will learn to shift from mental models dominated by events to models that recognize long-term patterns of change and the underlying structures that produce those patterns. Such a shift will reduce the "linear thinking" that dominates most decision-making mental models, and it will promote decisions based on shared understandings of interrelationships and patterns of change. And therein lies the path to *systems thinking*—the philosophical alternative to the pervasive reductionism in Western culture that seeks simple answers to complex questions.

Shared vision

A *shared vision* powerful influences organizational life. At its most basic level, it answers the question, "What do we want to create?" Shared visions derive from individuals' desire to connect with each other in important undertakings, and they create a sense of commonality that gives coherence to diverse activities. When employees truly share a vision, they connect—and their common aspiration binds them together.

Many shared visions are *extrinsic* (the attempt to gain ever larger markets, for example). But extrinsic visions, once achieved, can move an organization into a defensive posture ("Let's protect what we have.") *Intrinsic* visions, however, focus on inner standards of excellence and call forth the creativity and excitement associated with new programs and projects. Extrinsic and intrinsic visions can coexist, but sole reliance on an extrinsic vision can weaken an organization over time.

A shared vision changes employees' relationship to their organization. It promotes trust, courage, and a common identity—and it aligns individual and organizational goals. It helps establish an overarching goal that helps organizational members evaluate beliefs, strengths, and shortcomings—both individual and organizational. It promotes risk-taking and experimentation and counters strong status quo forces. And it answers management's question, "How can we foster long term commitment?"

Organizations that strive to build a shared vision continually encourage members to develop their *personal* visions. Without a personal vision, individuals simply "sign up" for someone else's vision. The result? Compliance instead of commitment. Personal mastery forms the foundation for a shared vision. Shared vision can generate levels of creative tension that go far beyond individuals' "comfort levels." And the greatest contributors to a lofty vision are those who can "hold" this creative tension—who can focus unwaveringly on the vision and steadily press their inquiry into current reality. These individuals, deeply convinced of their ability to create their future, contribute strongly to organizational life.

In building shared visions, managers and leaders first must abandon the notion that visions are passed down from "on high" or that they derive from an organization's institutionalized planning processes. Top-down, one-shot "visions" fail to build on personal visions and usually fail to "come alive." They fail to create energy and commitment—and they simply don't inspire. Moreover, a vision that is inconsistent with organizational members' values will not only fail to inspire genuine enthusiasm—it may foster outright cynicism. Vision becomes a living force only when people truly believe in their capacity to shape their future.

Many managers continue to insist that their problems are caused by people "out there" or by "the system." They pay lip service to a "can do" proactive approach and carefully avoid any suggestion that the organization can't create its future. Yet they persist in *reacting* to change—rather than *generating* change. This "event mentality" drives out real vision and leaves behind only empty "vision statements."

Team learning

Team learning—the process of aligning and developing the capacity of a team to create the results its members truly desire—builds on the discipline of shared vision. It also builds on the personal mastery discipline, since talented teams are composed of talented individuals. But shared vision and talent alone are insufficient. The world contains many talented individuals who share a vision for a while, yet ultimately fail to learn. Great symphony orchestras possess talent and a shared vision, but they also know how to *play together*—the critical element in their artistic success.

Team learning has three critical dimensions. First, teams must think insightfully about complex issues and harness the intelligence of the collective mind. Certain organizational forces—coercive power and excessive self-interest, for example—can reduce a team's effectiveness. But team members can learn to control deleterious forces.

Second, learning teams must take innovative, coordinated action. The championship sports teams and great jazz ensembles exemplify spontaneous yet coordinated modes of thought and action. Outstanding teams in organizations develop the same kind of relationship—"an operational trust" that allows each team member to act in ways that complement other team members' actions.

Third, a learning team understands the potential of its team members to influence other organizational members. And effective team members continually promote the practices and skills of team learning throughout the organization.

Team learning is a collective discipline that requires the skills of *dialogue* and *discussion*, the two distinct ways that teams converse. *In dialogue, individuals freely and creatively explore (brainstorm) complex and subtle issues; they listen deeply and suspend their own views. In discussion, individuals present and defend different views and search for the view that best supports potential decisions.*

Dialogue and discussion are potentially complementary activities, but most teams lack the ability to distinguish (and to move freely between) the two forms of communication. Effective learning teams acquire the ability to deal creatively with the powerful forces that oppose productive dialogue and discussion. They learn to recognize conflicting interests, and they find ways to negotiate "win-win" solutions.

Finally, team learning requires practice, an activity that many modern organizations fail to promote. Through practice and performance, team members find *alignment* and a common direction, purpose, and vision. They harmonize and conserve their energy. And they discover ways to complement each other's efforts without sacrificing their personal interests.

The team learning discipline remains poorly understood. Until we can more accurately describe the phenomenon, it will remain somewhat mysterious, and we will be unable to distinguish clearly between group intelligence and "groupthink"—the acquiescence to conformity. When we develop reliable methods for fostering group learning, we will take a critical step toward building learning organizations.

Systems thinking

Systems thinking, Senge's fifth discipline, integrates the other disciplines and fuses them into a coherent body of theory and practice. It helps organizational members see how the disciplines interrelate, and it reminds us that the whole can exceed the sum of its parts. (We will discuss systems thinking in chapter 9.)

Power, politics, and the learning organization

In an ideal world, all organizational groups would be described in terms such as *supportive, harmonious, trusting, collaborative, cooperative, and effective.* All organizational members would consistently promote the organization's interests. And no employees would withhold information, restrict output, attempt to "build empires," publicize their successes, hide their failures, distort performance figures, or in any other way engage in activities that promote only their self-interest.

In the real world, however, power and politics often defeat an organization's best attempts to develop shared values and to nurture a true learning environment. And a highly politicized organizational culture, inexorably grinding up the most worthy vision, can dissolve mutual commitment and block systemic change. Unfortunately, we too readily acquiesce to the insidious and deleterious influences of organizational politicking. We too quickly accept the arbitrary power and political machinations that promote an authoritarian organizational ethos. "You can't get away from politics," we say, as we steadily surrender our basic values and our hope for openness and freedom.

But we *can* break the grip of internal politics, and we *can* build organizational climates dominated not by power and politics but by profound knowledge (especially the ability to ask the right questions) and the disciplines of the learning organization. First, however, we must understand some dynamics of organizational power and politics—and the antidotes to them.

We convert power into influence through *systems of influence* that operate simultaneously and powerfully influence organizational life. The system of *authority* (formal power), the system of *ideology* (shared beliefs and values), the system of *expertise* (knowledge and skills), and the system of *politics* (political games) all combine to convert power into influence. But it is the system of politics that we often find most troubling and unsettling.

Politics

Stephen Robbins defines politics as ". . . any behavior by an organizational member that is self-serving." It is *functional*, he says, when the behavior assists in the maintenance of the organization's goals. It is *dysfunctional* when it hinders those goals.[3] An organization's politics can be seen most clearly in the conflicts and power plays that sometimes occupy center stage—and in the countless interpersonal intrigues that pervade organizational life in less obvious ways. And we can analyze organizational politics by focusing on relations between and among *interest*, *conflict*, and *power* principles.

Interests

Interests involve a complex set of predispositions that embrace our goals, values, desires, and expectations and that influence our behavior. We tend to view our interests as *areas of concern* that need to be preserved or enlarged. We live in the midst of our interests, and we readily defend them and fight to maintain and strengthen them.

We bring our *task interests* (concepts about the work we perform), our *career interests* (visions about our individual futures), and our *extramural interests* (views about our lives outside the organization) into an organizational setting. These interests shape our approaches to our jobs and careers, and the tensions between and among them render our relation to work inherently political.

Organizational members possess differing interests and frequently desire different courses of action. These differences create a tension that the organization attempts to resolve in a number of ways: 1) autocratically ("We'll do it this way."), 2) bureaucratically ("We're supposed to do it this way."), or 3) democratically ("How shall we do it?"). In each case, the choice between alternative paths of action usually hinges on the power relations between and among the actors involved. By focusing on how divergent *interests* give rise to conflicts (visible and invisible)—and by understanding ways individuals frequently act only in their self-interest (often at the expense of the organization's interest)—we can analyze organizational politics as rigorously as we analyze any other form of organizational behavior.

The sociologist Tom Burns notes that most modern organizations are designed as systems of simultaneous competition and collaboration, and they inevitably promote various kinds of politicking. One needn't be consciously cunning or deviously political to end up playing organizational politics. Political behavior is a fairly natural response to the conflict and tension that divergent interests create.

But when we understand that organizational politicking grows out of diverse interests (to which conflicts merely lend visible form), then we possess a means for penetrating beneath the surface of any conflict and understanding its genesis. When we understand the potential for conflict among interests, we find a means for decoding the personal agendas that underlie specific actions—and, more important, we discover ways to understand political behavior and reduce destructive politicking.

Conflict

We frequently attribute organizational conflict to some regrettable set of circumstances. ("It's a personality problem." "They're rivals who always meet head-on." "Those two groups never get along.") The real roots of conflict, however, run deeper. *Conflict arises when interest collide*—and we usually can trace organizational conflict to some perceived or real divergence of *interests*.

We tend to view conflict as an unfortunate event that we'd just as soon avoid. If we accept, however, that organizational members promote differing interests, then we can view conflict as inevitable—and even as a positive element that energizes the organization and alerts it to possibilities for new opportunities. When we focus on the divergent *interests* that give rise to conflicts (implicit and explicit), we begin to see the sources of political strategies and power plays. When we understand how divergent interests contribute to conflict, we find resolutions that hinge not on power plays but on negotiations that respect separate interests—

and that help organizations and individuals in conflict achieve their separate interests.

Conflict is a growth industry. More and more conflicts require negotiation. In their book *Getting to Yes: Negotiating Agreement Without Giving In*, Fisher and Ury set forth a principle (developed at the Harvard Negotiation Project) they call *principled negotiation*.[4] The principled negotiation method is hard on the merits and soft on the people, and it provides some valuable techniques for negotiating agreement.

Power

Organizations can be viewed as decision-making systems. And individuals who possess the ability to shape decision processes powerfully influence organizational affairs. Decision-making power involves control of three interrelated elements: decision *premises*, decision *processes*, and decision *issues* and *objectives*.

Much of the political activity within an organization revolves around the control of agendas and other decision *premises* that influence the approach to a specific decision. By thwarting or avoiding explicit discussion of an issue, an individual may prevent a core issue from even surfacing—and, thus, maintain the status quo.

Control of decision *processes*, usually more obvious than the control of decision premises, involves the ability to influence 1) how a decision should be made, 2) who should make it, and 3) when it will be made. Organizational members can promote or block a proposed course of action by manipulating the ground rules that guide decision making.

An organizational member can also influence *issues* and *objectives* by emphasizing the importance of particular constraints, by selecting and evaluating the alternatives, and by highlighting the importance of certain values or outcomes. An individual's eloquence, command of the facts, passionate commitment, or sheer tenacity and endurance can help him or her influence decisions.

Politics and culture are inherent features of organizational life. Organizational members must guard against the danger of seeing politics and hidden agendas at every turn. But the model of *interest, conflict,* and *power* described here provides a practical and systematic means for understanding the relation between politics and organizational life—and for seeing the key role that power plays in determining political outcomes. (We'll have more to say about power in Chapter 10.)

Politics and health care organizations

Health care organizations coordinate the activities of a diverse group of individuals—including highly trained medical professionals and other nonmedical professionals (administrators, for example). Medical organizations, like other organizations, convert power into influence through *authority* (formal power), *ideology* (shared beliefs and values), *expertise* (knowledge and skills), and *politics* (political games). In many health organizations, influence systems traditionally have been based on expertise rather than on authority. But varying interests also collide within health care organizations, and *politics* can operate powerfully for various reasons:

1) Health care goals may be difficult to define—and professional performance difficult to measure. When health care administrators attempt to impose standards and criteria on medical professionals, interests may conflict—and professionals may easily deflect the standards.

2) Health care professionals may identify more strongly with their discipline than with the organization. With the presence of many professional groups in an organization, interests may vary—and intergroup conflict and factions may develop.

3) Health care professionals tend to focus on their own skill development rather than on broad organizational goals. Although the skills are well-defined, the circumstances in which they are applied are less clearly-defined—and territorial disputes (turf fights) over patients, clients, and activities may develop among the various disciplines and specialties.

4) Health care professionals give highest priority to the needs of their patients and often come into conflict with managers and others who attempt to advance organization-wide goals.

These organizational characteristics—together with two divergent power structures (the "medical professional" and the "formal administrative")—can generate ambiguity and conflict. And they can foster a political climate in which professionals compete for resources and attempt to advance only their self-interest. When organizations attempt strategic changes, power often gets redistributed, and decision-making processes sometimes lose structure. Individuals and groups with conflicting interests may then attempt to mobilize resources and vanquish each other—usually to the organization's disadvantage.

Learning organizations understand that politics operates in all forms of organizational life and that certain forms of legitimate politicking are appropriate and necessary. Learning organizations, however, also recognize that most people prefer to avoid political game playing—and the perversions that accompany it. And they motivate their members to look beyond individual interests to the common good.

Conclusion

Learning organizations challenge old mental models and promote the common visions and values that move people beyond self-interest. They use conflict in ways that enhance creative tension and innovation. And they build skills and capabilities that deepen confidence and enhance true learning. These capabilities fall into three natural categories.

Aspiration. All the learning disciplines help individuals, teams, and organizations achieve their true objectives. But the disciplines of personal mastery and shared vision play critical roles in developing organizational learning and change capabilities.

Personal mastery flourishes in an organizational culture that encourages personal vision development and a commitment to truth. Many practices that promote personal mastery are associated with the other disciplines—with the ability 1) to develop a more systemic worldview, 2) to reflect on tacit assumptions (mental models), 3) to express one's vision and to respect other perspectives, and 4) to explore others' view of current reality. Successful personal mastery programs strive to develop the other four individual disciplines (systems thinking, mental models, shared vision, team learning) in concert. But they strive also to integrate the disciplines and to discover the ways they enhance and support each other. Effective mastery programs also maintain freedom and choice—and avoid compulsory programs.

A personal and collective vision greatly promotes personal mastery. And generative learning—the ability to expand one's ability to create—usually remains an abstract and meaningless principle without the lift of a vivid and compelling vision. The power of fear drives negative visions, and fear can produce significant short-term changes. But the power of aspiration drives positive visions—and aspiration provides a continuing source of learning and growth.

Reflection and conversation. The ability to reflect on deep assumptions and patterns—to surface, test, and improve our "mental models"—represents a powerful tool for change. Our mental models influence not only our perceptions (what we see) but also our actions (what we do), and successful learning organizations strive always to help employees reflect on their mental models and articulate their perceptions.

Effective learning organization members also develop the ability to engage in team learning and "learningful conversation." And they acquire the ability to engage in dialogue—an activity that assumes a free flow of meaning between people and the capacity to access a larger "pool of common meaning."

Conceptualization. Conceptualization skills provide the ability to see larger patterns and to identify relationships—to engage, that is, in systems thinking. When we challenge our mental models and then integrate a systems perspective into our worldview, we fundamentally alter our thinking. We move away from language designed to address simple static problems—and toward language designed to confront complex, dynamic realities. And we engage in systems thinking—a powerful tool for change and innovation.

REFERENCES

1. Peter Senge, *The Fifth Discipline: The Art & Practice of the Learning Organization* (New York: Doubleday, 1990).
2. George Bernard Shaw, epistle dedicatory for *Man and Superman* (London, 1903).
3. Stephen Robbins, *Organizational Behavior: Concepts, Controversies, and Applications* (Englewood Cliffs NJ: Prentice Hall, 1989), 4.
4. William Ury, *Getting to Yes: Negotiating Agreement Without Giving In* (New York: Penguin Books, 1983).

SUGGESTED READINGS

Peter Senge, *The Fifth Discipline: The Art & Practice of the Learning Organization* (New York: Doubleday, 1990).
Peter Senge et al., *The Fifth Discipline Fieldbook: Strategies and Tools for Building a Learning Organization* (New York: Doubleday, 1994).
Chris Agyris, *Overcoming Organizational Defenses* (New York: Prentice-Hall, 1990).
Chris Agyris, *Strategy, Change, and Defensive Routines* (Boston: Pitman, 1985).
Gareth Morgan, *Images of Organizations* (Newbury Park CA: Sage Publications, 1986).

9

Health Care and Systems Thinking

Our health care system, a disparate collection of services, programs, and organizations, defies our best attempts to see it whole. We strain to see the "big picture," and when we fail, we focus our attentions on isolated parts and lose our connection to the whole.

Systems thinking provides the tools for seeing wholes *and* interlocking parts—and for comprehending underlying structures, relationships, patterns, and processes. Systems thinking helps us understand the subtle interconnections between and among family, organizational, and community systems that give the health care system its unique character. It provides the incentives and the means for integrating the other learning disciplines—*personal mastery, mental models, shared vision*, and *team learning*. And it offers an antidote to the sense of helplessness we often feel in this "age of interdependence."

We have created more information than we can absorb. We have fostered more interdependency than we can manage. And we have developed more complexity than we can understand. But these forces needn't overwhelm us. We needn't continue to fight complexity with complexity, devising increasingly complex (detailed) solutions to increasingly "complex" problems. Instead we can use systems thinking 1) to see interrelationships rather than linear cause and effect chains and 2) to perceive processes rather than "snapshots."

Before examining some specific elements of systems thinking, let's look briefly at a few ways that "old thinking" and outdated, deeply ingrained mental models interfere with the acquisition and development of a systems perspective.

Reductionism

The mechanistic or Newtonian view of reality, a paradigm that has dominated Western thought for 300 years, holds that the universe is indeed a huge mechanical system—and that complex phenomena (and systems) can be understood by 1) reducing them to their basic building blocks and then 2) examining the mechanisms through which the blocks or parts interact.

Reductionism has served us well in certain disciplines. In the biological sciences, for example, the reductionist approach has helped us understand cell biology, the nature of genes, and other scientific phenomena. But reductionist thinking has also imposed serious limits on our ability to analyze and understand (and change) human systems—including the organizations and institutions that deliver health care and other social goods and services.

The limitations surrounding the reductionist view has led (in part) to a more "complex" or "organic" paradigm that views the universe as a harmonious and indivisible whole—a network of dynamic relationships that includes human observers (and their consciousnesses) and that requires a *systems thinking* approach to institutional transformation, organizational change, and other earthly activities.

Systems thinking, *a discipline for seeing wholes*, provides an alternative to the pervasive reductionism in Western culture. Systems thinking seeks to move individuals and organizations toward "process" thinking. And it provides a conceptual framework, a body of knowledge, and a set of analytic tools for illuminating the full *patterns* in a system—and then helping us change them. Systems thinking leads us away from reductionism (with its inherent resistance to integrative concepts) and away also from linear thinking—another major impediment to seeing "wholes."

Linear thinking

We tend to think linearly—in terms of cause and effect. That is, we think that A influences B, and B influences C, and so on. Systems thinking, however, radically alters that view. *Systems thinking holds that every influence is both cause and effect—nothing is ever influenced in just one direction.* So, when A influences B, B also influences A—and both continually interrelate with C and D. And, thus, the circle of influence begins.

Every circle tells a story. By tracing the flows of influence, we begin to see a specific pattern (or patterns) of behavior—and the ways that pattern might be influenced. We see *circles of causality* (or influence). And when we move away from linear thinking and begin to see *circles of influence* rather than straight lines, we break out of our reactive mindsets and begin to think *systemically*. We see the mental models that trap us in outdated paradigms—and we begin to use creative tension in ways that help us shape our future.

When we begin to think systematically, we see the ways we influence our reality—and the ways our reality influences us. In addition, we abandon the notion that individuals create organizational and systemic problems. We give up the search for scapegoats and see more clearly that *all* system members share responsibility for system-generated outputs. Eventually, systems thinking forms a rich language that helps us describe a vast array of interrelationships and patterns of change. Ultimately, it simplifies life by helping us see the deeper (often hidden) patterns that lie behind events and details.

Systems thinking can be applied to all the activities associated with the maintenance and improvement of health care—including all the social actions and policies that contribute to our overall health status. But since most changes in the health care system will occur initially at the organizational level, we're mainly interested here in the ways systems thinking influences processes and roles within organizations. But what is an organization? And what are the basic system dynamics that influence organizational life—for better or for worse?

Organizational roles, processes, functions, and tasks

An organization has been defined as a system of roles (the structure of an organization) and a stream of activities (a set of organizational processes) designed to achieve shared goals. Roles and processes comprise the basic building blocks of an organization. The pattern or dynamic relationships among roles and the interrelationships between and among the processes make an organization a system rather than a random collection of interrelated (or unrelated) parts.

A *role* is simply the set of behaviors an organizational member is *expected* to perform and that he or she feels *obligated* to perform. A role combines the cumulative formal, informal, technical, and personal expectations about a job. *Role perception* relates to the way one sees the role, and *role performance* relates to the way one behaves in the role. Roles also contain *functions* (major domains of activity within the role) and *tasks* (specific activities used to carry out a function).

Roles do not provide us with set, rigid scripts. The fluidity of organizational life and the changing stream of activities in daily work life continually compel us to change our expectations (for ourselves and others) and, consequently, to redefine our roles and modify our behavior. To see an organization in terms of roles, however, helps us *begin* to see the patterns that underlie organizational activity.

These patterns consist largely of *functions* and *tasks* (but mainly tasks) that are linked together into *processes*. A process, in turn, consists of a set of inputs (including a sequence of tasks) that contribute to the delivery of a specific service or the manufacture of a certain product. Organizational work proceeds through stages within a process—and we can identify many processes within an organization.

When we begin to see processes as a series of related tasks and inputs—and then to see organizational work as a set of interrelated processes—we develop a clearer picture of organizational activity and a common (and more comprehensible) language for analyzing and discussing organizational issues. We develop the ability to define starting and ending points in a process, and we learn to ask important questions. What do we want from this process? What are the inputs (people, methods, machines, materials, measurements, and environmental factors), and how can changes in any of them enhance quality and efficiency? Which tasks are necessary along the process? Which can be eliminated or improved?

If a set of inputs and a series of tasks can be called a *process*, then a group of related processes can be called a *system*. And our attempts to change systems, especially large systems, often frustrate (even defeat) us. Most systems change slowly—and large systems usually change exceedingly slowly.

When we focus on processes, however, we gain the ability to identify specific steps and related inputs within the process, and we begin to understand where and how those steps and inputs fit into the total process. When we see clearly a process, we understand how it relates to other processes and how it fits into the larger picture—the system. When we see both the larger picture and the interlocking parts, *we are engaging in systems thinking*. And when we view a system as a set of interrelated processes, we see the system's architecture—and we discover opportunities for improving the system through improving individual processes. Moreover, we begin to discover separate but interrelated systems between and among organizations. And we develop the ability to draw boundaries around various systems and sub-systems.

We expend enormous amounts of time and energy attempting to make wholesale changes to the health care "system." But its magnitude and complexity (and the difficulty of even defining it) defy our attempts to see it whole and to prescribe macro changes that will produce predictable results. But we needn't think only in terms of macro system changes. Indeed, attempts to see the entire health care system as a coherent entity may prove not only frustrating but also ultimately unproductive. Perhaps, instead, we need to "think globally and act locally." Margaret Wheatley puts it this way:

> I believe the evolving emphasis in our society to "think globally, act locally" expresses a quantum perception of reality. Acting locally is a sound strategy for changing large systems. Instead of trying to map an elaborate system, the advice is to work with the system that you know, one you can get your arms around. If we look at this strategy with Newtonian eyes, we would say that we are creating incremental change. Little by little, system by system, we develop enough momentum to affect the larger society.
>
> A quantum view would explain the success of these efforts differently. Acting locally allows us to work with the movement and flow of simultaneous events within that small system. We are more likely to become synchronized with that system, and thus to have an impact. These changes in small places, however, create large-systems change, not because they build one upon the other, but because they share in the unbroken wholeness that has united them all along. Our activities in one part of the whole create nonlocal causes that emerge far from us. There is value in working with the system any place it manifests because unseen connections will create effects at a distance, in places we never thought. This model of change—of small starts, surprises, unseen connections, quantum leaps—matches our experience more closely than our favored models of incremental change.[1]

Margaret Wheatley makes a strong case for 1) analyzing work *processes* within organizations, 2) examining relationships between and among processes (both within and outside the organization), and 3) studying the relationships among health care organizations along the continuum of care. When we apply systems thinking to this scale of activity, we begin to see processes and patterns. We reduce our tendency toward reductionist and linear thinking, and we position ourselves to find unlimited opportunities for change and reform at a level we can understand and effect.

Let's look briefly at a few more key systems concepts and their relation to organizational change and innovation.

Boundaries

Boundaries have been defined as lines that fix "a limit or extent," and all systems possess a boundary. A boundary indicates a specific "domain of analysis" and marks off one territory from another. And system boundaries serve important purposes.

First, boundaries create a sense of identity; they help us distinguish one entity or system from another. Boundaries may be arbitrarily drawn in some cases. But they help us define a system, and they serve as devices for engaging (and discussing) the boundaries of other systems.

Second, boundaries (ambiguous though they are at times) help us make decisions about the level and scale of our change efforts. Should we, for example, attempt to change the entire health care system (an unlikely prospect at best). Or should we focus our activities on community-wide change? Or on change within organizations—or units within organizations? Any useful system change dialogue must begin with some agreement about the the system's dimensions.

Third, boundaries help us understand the interconnectedness between and among systems—and the need to establish effective "structural interactions" throughout the broad system. Cooperative interactions among various systems lie at the heart of effective organizational, institutional, and social change activities. But effective cooperation rests heavily on the ability to define so-called "autonomous" systems—and then establish agreements between and among them.

Reinforcing loops

Reinforcing and balancing loops constitute two of the most basic building blocks in systems representations. Reinforcing loops generate exponential growth and collapse. They promote growth—but they also may accelerate decline. In a reinforcing process, a small change builds on itself, and a small action snowballs—sometimes into a "vicious cycle" (when things go from bad to worse) and sometimes into a "virtuous cycle" (when things steadily improve).

Reinforcing loops (or amplifying processes) create a snowball effect, and they can powerfully influence the success or failure of all systems—including organizations. When organizational members remark that "We're on a roll" or (conversely) "We're going to hell in a handbasket," they're probably caught up in a reinforcing loop.

But pure accelerating growth or decline patterns rarely continue unchecked. Certain *balancing loops* slow, stop, divert, and even reverse their progress.

Balancing loops

Nature loves a balance. Individuals, organizations, and societies all possess balancing mechanisms that maintain stability and equilibrium—and that help them adjust to environmental changes. The human body, for example, contains thousands of balancing mechanisms that maintain temperature, blood pressure, and other functions. Organizations also contain balancing loops that help them adapt to their environments and stay within their "natural" operating range.

Thus, when organizational members say "We're running into walls" or "We can't break through the barrier," there's probably a balancing loop nearby. Balancing loops often engender frustration, but they also serve valuable purposes. They slow or stop runaway vicious cycles, for example, and they provide self-correcting and self-regulating mechanisms.

Balancing loops are always bound to a target—a constraint or goal that is often set by the system's forces. That is, when current reality fails to match the balancing loop's target, the resultant gap (between the target and the system's actual performance) generates pressure that the system cannot ignore. The greater the gap, the greater the pressure. The system seems to know "how things ought to be," and it seeks a return to "normalcy."

Thus, the first step in understanding the behavior of a balancing loop is to recognize the gap between target and performance—and then to identify the goal or constraint that drives it. But goals may be hidden, and managers and other organizational members may not be able to identify readily the forces impeding productivity.

Hidden goals

All organizations and institutions possess goals—usually explicitly stated. But organizations frequently respond to *implicit* or *hidden* goals that can frustrate efforts to achieve announced objectives. Certain stated quality goals, for example, may be thwarted by unannounced profitability goals. When organizational goals are *explicit* and generally congruent with members' individual goals, the organization tends to move steadily toward its stated objective. *Implicit* (unstated and hidden) goals, however, call forth *balancing loops* that are difficult to detect and that insidiously impede progress toward explicit goals.

These balancing loops resist change, and the resistance often seems to come from nowhere—but it has a real source. It represents the organization's attempt to maintain a *hidden system goal*, and it arises out of a threat to traditional norms and usual ways of doing business. An organization that is "running hard just to stay in one place" is probably laboring under the restraints of a hidden goal. Effective leaders and managers don't attempt to overpower resistance. Rather, they find the source of the resistance—the *hidden goal*—and clear the path to explicit organizational goals.

Delays

Delays constitute another major element in systems thinking. And they occur often in both reinforcing and balancing loops. A delay represents the gap in time between an intervention and the consequences of the intervention. And delays can powerfully influence a system. We all experience and expect delays: we invest today with the hope of a payoff tomorrow. But in organizational life, we often fail to recognize or understand the inevitable (sometimes necessary) delay between action and results. And when we fail to perceive the intended consequences of our intervention, we sometimes take aggressive and unnecessary action to force change. We "overshoot."

For example, when we attempt to increase the water temperature in a shower that contains a ten-second delay, we may think our initial action had no consequence. We adjust, but then we often "overshoot" in the hot water direction. When we feel the gush of overly hot water, we "overshoot" in the other direction—the cold water direction. And on and on we go through the balancing loop process Each adjustment cycle compensates somewhat for the previous cycle. But the more aggressively we act, the longer it takes to reach the desired temperature. We don't take into account *delay*, and we unnecessarily intervene. We "teeter-totter" around a desired level—and we unnecessarily oscillate the system.

At the organizational level, these unneeded interventions (based usually on our linear thinking) delude us into believing we are taking effective action. They also can produce unintended consequences, and they may generate instablity. Most important, they frequently thwart an organization's ability to find efficiencies and opportunities that provide *long-term* payoffs. When addressing special and common causes of variation within a process, managers must allow time for the interventions to make their full impact and for the process to restabilize. Managers who recognize the delay phenomenon avoid unnecessary interventions and ultimately (with patience) improve the quality of the output.

Complexity

Sophisticated analytic tools and elegant strategic plans often fail to produce dramatic breakthroughs—or any results at all. Our best change efforts fall victim to indiscernible problems buried deep within the organization's work *processes*. Even when we can't see the source of the problem, we may see the *complexity* the problem generates—as the process or system attempts to compensate for the problem. And in the face of overwhelming complexity, we often despair and ask ourselves: "How can we possibly cope with such complexity?" "How can we figure it all out?" We *can* learn to address complexity and enhance quality and efficiency, but first we need to distinguish between two types of complexity—*detail* and *dynamic* complexity.

Detail complexity

Detail complexity refers to the many *variables* within a process. We encounter detail complexity when we mix ingredients into a pizza or assemble a complicated machine—or engage in other work activities that involve numerous variables. Unfortunately, most "system analyses" focus on these variables—on the complex array of details that distract us from seeing the major *patterns* and *interrelationships* that influence outcomes and that frequently defeat our attempts to find comprehensive, rational explanations.

Detail complexity manifests itself when managers and employees attempt to improve a process without addressing the patterns and relationships within the process. They address one variable in the process—an action that only distorts other parts of the process and frequently creates more problems in other areas. Managers captured by this problem-solving approach continue to add steps and ultimately wind up treating only the symptoms of the underlying problems. They fail to address all the factors that contribute to the outcome. They fail, that is, to think systemically, and they fall victim to *detail complexity*.

We possess enormous capacities to handle detail complexity. We learn to drive cars and play music—tasks that involve hundreds of variables and require rapid changes and instant responses. Some part of our human mind is designed to deal with detail complexity, and many problems can be resolved through addressing detail complexity.

Dynamic complexity

Most major problems, however, require the ability to address *dynamic complexity*—the patterns and interrelationships between and among processes and systems. In dynamic complexity, cause and effect don't readily reveal themselves, and the effects of interventions are difficult to discern. Systems thinking is designed for dynamic complexity. Systems thinking helps us see *through* detail complexity into the underlying dynamics and interactions that generate change. And it organizes complexity into a coherent story that reveals the greatest opportunities for change and innovation. When we see the interactions between and among inputs and the reciprocal flows of influence within a process—the *dynamic complexity*—we discover solutions to seemingly intractable problems. And we begin to understand the nature of *variation* in a process.

Some managers (trapped by their linear thinking) react to any kind of variation, and sometimes their intervention provides an immediate and visible payoff. Often, however, their intervention interferes with a more important task—developing consistent and clear methods for analyzing processes, understanding dynamic interrelationships, and then reducing or eliminating the *root causes* of variation in a product or service. When we understand the nature of variation, we equip ourselves with a powerful tool for improving efficiency and outcomes.

Variation

Traditional health care quality assurance (QA) efforts have depended on compliance audits, motivation programs, and other dubious tools. These QA efforts have focused on observed outcomes and non-conforming "outliers" and have attempted to sort out the "poor" performers from the "good" performers.

The more recent continuous quality improvement (CQI) approaches differ significantly from traditional QA concepts. CQI views health care and other services as a set of *processes* that leads to an *output*. CQI searches for opportunities to improve the *processes*—and thus reduce variation in the outputs (services, products) of those processes.

In a health care organization, these processes work together to deliver care. And the quality of that care depends on the quality of the *inputs* into the processes—on the people, methods, machines, materials, measurements, and environmental factors that surround health care. Changes in any of these inputs will affect the degree of variation and the quality of the services.

- *People*. Differences in education, training, and experience among organizational members inevitably introduces variation into a process.
- *Methods*. Differences in policies and procedures— and differences in their application—can influence service and product variation.

- *Machines and materials.* Differences in the ability of the machines and materials to carry out their function cause variation.
- *Measurements.* Differences in the criteria used to measure outcomes, together with varying applications of the criteria, introduce variation into the outcome data.
- *Environment.* Differences in the various service environments (e.g., nursing homes, clinics, hospitals) and in the community and social environment influence service variation.

Systems thinkers use analytic (as opposed to enumerative) statistics to assess the *stability* of a process and to measure the variations in its outputs. And they frequently use a control chart, an analytic tool developed by Walter Shewart, to help them monitor processes and assess outcomes. Using various information collection methods, process analysts gather outcome data over time and chart the results on a control chart. They then use statistical methods to establish the mean or median of the data—and then to establish the upper and lower control limits of the output data.

Control charts tell managers and other organizational members when a process is in a stable state—when, that is, the process is in a state of statistical control and thus producing predictable outputs. In a stable process, the variation in the output data will fall randomly within the established limits of the control chart. But since process inputs (people, education, methods, machines, materials, measurements, and environmental factors) vary, process outputs will also inevitably vary to some degree. And although managers and employees must strive continuously to reduce variation, a "zero defect" state (complete elimination of output variation) will always remain unattainable. Indeed, relentless pursuit of such a goal—reflecting an inability to accept some normal variation—can prove unacceptably time-consuming and costly.

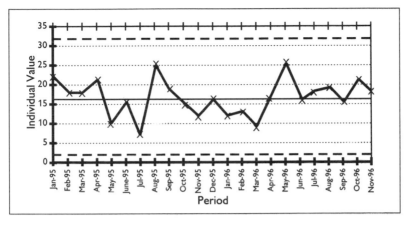

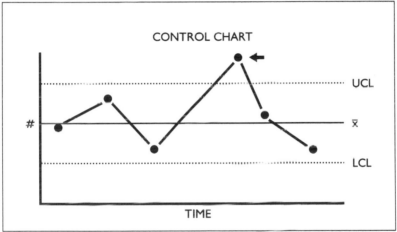

Two examples of control charts

In many cases, managers and other employees use intuition and common sense to eliminate obvious causes of variation and to bring the process into statistical control—into a state of predictability. As Deming points out, however, a "worker, when he has reached statistical control, has put into the process all that he has to offer." Without management support, workers cannot by themselves move to the second step—improving process ouputs by reducing *common causes* of variation.

When control charts show that the process outputs are beyond the control limits—or consistently above or below the established median—managers may fairly conclude that a special cause (a special occurrence or event) has precipitated a change in the previously stable process. Therefore, workers and managers must analyze the data and the process—and then attempt to identify (and eliminate) the *special cause* and to restabilize the process. Deming estimates, however, that only six percent of process problems can be attributed to special causes of variation—the other 94 percent of opportunities for process improvement lie within the *process and system design*.

Management, says Deming, must provide the skills and organizational environment that allow employees to identify and reduce (or eliminate) *special causes of variation*—and thus keep outputs predictable. In addition, TQM managers must also "empower" employees with the authority and ability to identify *common causes of variation* —the source of most outcome variation. When all organizational members work to identify common causes of variation, they operate out of the central CQI idea— managers and other employees improve output through continuously improving processes.

Toward that end, employees must understand the nature and function of measurement systems—one of the most essential process inputs. In the words of Sashkin and Kiser:

> Measurement systems designed to support TQM must be focused on improvement of processes, not on control of those responsible for work processes. This means emphasizing process metrics, not results metrics. The aim is to assess and improve work processes by identifying and correcting factors that cause undesired variation. This is very different from the notion of controlling *people*. The way in which measurement systems are designed and used determines whether employees support or subvert a TQM effort.[2]

When we recognize that we improve quality through reducing variation, we begin to understand that it is the imperfect processes that mainly contribute to outcome variations. And, since employees presumably perform as well as the process allows, we ask some central questions. Do organizational members possess the methods, machines, materials, measurements, environments, knowledge, and skills that will allow them to achieve individual and organizational objectives? How do we measure variation? *And how do we determine when and whether we should take corrective action?*

Many managers attempt to improve quality by adjusting (and overadjusting) stable processes. They treat common causes of variation as special causes and "tamper" with the process. And when we tamper with a stable process in statistical control, we often increase variation, defects, and mistakes. But when we learn to distinguish between special and common causes of variation, we take a long step toward learning how and when to intervene in a process. And we begin to understand the critical principle of *leverage.*

Leverage

Leverage—the ability to see where and how specific actions can effect the most significant, enduring changes—contributes powerfully to process improvement. Effective leverage follows a basic principle: the best results derive not from large-scale efforts but from small well-focused, well-placed actions. And these highly-targeted, effective actions offer some tremendous opportunities for change and innovation at the organizational level and across the continuum of care.

Our nonsystemic ways of thinking, however, frequently lead us into low-leverage (unproductive) change efforts. We focus on areas that show the greatest stress, and we repair or ameliorate the symptoms. We find short-term solutions that sometimes hurt us in the long-term. *And we fail to find the leverage point that can provide the highest return with the least effort.*

Moreover, the obvious leverage points tend to be the wrong ones. High leverage points easily elude us, and we waste our resources chasing phantoms. In addition, when we find a high leverage point and apply the correct and effective action, we often find that things tend to get worse before they get better (just as they initially seem to get better when we're working on the wrong leverage point—and treating only symptoms). True change opportunities usually don't reveal themselves readily, and the high leverage point may be far removed from the problem or symptoms of the problem.

There are no simple rules for finding high-leverage points, but there are ways of thinking that can improve change prospects. Effective managers and leaders will avoid tampering with stable systems. They will identify first the high leverage point and then determine the kind of change that can produce lasting significant improvement with minimal effort. And they will continually and continuously seek out high-leverage opportunities.

Laws of the Fifth Discipline

In his book *The Fifth Discipline: The Art & Practice of the Learning Discipline*, Peter Senge summarizes some basic systems thinking principles, and a brief review can perhaps help us internalize these powerful concepts.[3]

1) *See interrelationships—avoid "snapshot thinking."* We've been conditioned to see the world in static images. We must learn to see interrelationships and circles of causality rather than linear cause-effect chains. We must learn to see processes rather than snapshots.

2) *Move beyond blame.* When we see an organizational problem, we tend to blame external events or incompetent and unmotivated employees. We must learn that there is no "outside"—there is no cause and effect. We are all part of a single system. And we must learn to recognize change opportunities within organizational processes and systems.

3) *Differentiate between detail complexity and dynamic complexity.* Some types of complexity are strategically more important than others. Effective leverage lies in understanding dynamic complexity—in seeing the major patterns and interrelationships that underlie the variation in the process outputs.

4) *Find the right leverage point.* Systems thinking teaches us that small, well-focused, well-placed actions can produce significant, enduring improvements—although initially they may seem to make things worse. We must learn to identify high leverage points—points at which small, low-effort actions produce lasting, significant improvements.

5) *Avoid symptomatic solutions.* Linear thinking often leads to interventions that focus on symptoms rather than underlying causes. We gain temporary relief, but we create pressures for still more low-leverage (unproductive) interventions—and we lose the ability to address fundamental problems. We must learn to avoid quick fixes that lead us into an endless spiral of low-leverage, unproductive interventions.

6) *Accept delay.* When managers intervene in a system, they must allow time for the system to stabilize before they apply more corrective action. Managers often underestimate the time required for the process to stabilize, and they often "overshoot." They apply aggressive and unnecessary action to hasten progress, but their actions delay the necessary stabilization—and slow progress. We must learn to accept delays and to recognize the natural pace of change efforts.

7) *Maintain standards and goals.* We must not only avoid quick fixes—we must also hold to our performance standards. When we sacrifice quality and stan-

dards to achieve short-term goals, we ultimately sacrifice our ability to grow and achieve long-term goals.

8) *Look for "win-win" solutions.* Individuals and organizations often attempt to increase their welfare and security by dominating their competition. But when one side gets ahead, the other side feels threatened and aggressively retaliates—and an escalating cycle begins. This cycle often goes way beyond anyone's expectation or wish. We must learn to identify and establish collaboration strategies that help both sides "win."

9) *Manage the commons.* We often use a commonly available but limited resource solely for individual needs. We gain initial rewards, but eventually we either erode or entirely deplete our resource base— and sacrifice the common good. Individual needs must be balanced against broad socials needs. We must learn to "manage our commons" through education, self-regulation, peer pressure, and official regulating mechanisms (ideally designed by participants).

10) *Recognize that the harder one pushes, the harder the system pushes back.* Well-intentioned interventions often call forth responses from the system that offset the intervention's benefits. Systems thinkers call this phenomenon *compensating feedback*. When our initial efforts fail to produce lasting results, we often "push harder," convinced that greater effort will produce desired results. All this effort, however, may blind us to the ways we are contributing to the obstacles. We must quit "pushing" and look for fundamental, systemic obstacles to change.

11) *Recognize that the easy way out usually leads back in.* We apply familiar solutions to problems. We stick to tactics and strategies we understand, and we keep

pushing them—even while fundamental problems persist and worsen. We look for a "bigger hammer" to drive home our outdated solutions—instead of questioning our mental models and looking for new solutions that will help us solve new problems.

12) *Recognize that faster is slower*. Virtually all natural systems, including organizations, grow at an optimal rate, and that rate is far less than the fastest possible growth. Excessive growth will slow down an operation. Systems principles don't serve as excuses for inaction. To speed progress, however, we must look for a new type of action rooted in a new way of thinking—*systems thinking*.

Systems thinking and health care reform

The American health care system looks like a "non-system" until we try to change it. And then we learn even more about the system's complexity and intricate pattern of relationships—among patients, patients' family members, multiple providers, multiple organizations, payment systems, resources, service and product ideas, managerial beliefs and attitudes, and hundreds of other elements.

When we attempt to change system components, we tend to intervene at the level of rules, physical structure, work processes, material and information flows, reward systems, control systems, and other domains where the elements are more visible and the solutions more apparent. The systems perspective, however, teaches us to look for deep-seated values, attitudes, beliefs—and *multiple levels of explanation*.

In our change efforts, we often direct attention only to the first level—*to events*—and we trap ourselves in reactive stances. When we focus on the second level—*on behavior patterns*—we begin to see long-term trends and to assess their implications, and we begin to break the reactive grip. But when we focus on the third level—*on system explanations*—we ask the critical question. What causes the behavior patterns? And we begin to discover the underlying causes of behavior patterns at a level they can be changed. We begin, that is, to challenge our mental models and to engage in *systems thinking.*

Systems thinking gives us the problem-solving tools and the language we need to augment and change the usual ways we talk about complex health issues. It helps us see interdependencies across the continuum of care and the need for collaboration between and among health organizations. And it can help us promote the creative and lasting change we need to meet the health care challenges of the coming century.

REFERENCES

1. Margaret Wheatley, *Leadership and the New Science* (San Francisco: Berrett-Koehler, 1994), 42–43.
2. Marshall Sashkin and Kenneth Kiser, *Putting Total Quality Management to Work* (San Francisco: Berret-Koehler, 1993), 80.
3. Peter Senge, *The Fifth Discipline: The Art & Practice of the Learning Organization* (New York: Doubleday, 1990), 57–67.

SUGGESTED READINGS

D. Balestracci and J. Barlow, *Quality Improvement: Practical Applications in Medical Group Practice* (Englewood CO: Center for Research in Ambulatory Health Care Administration, 1996).

Draper Kauffman, Jr., *Systems 1: An Introduction to Systems Thinking* (Minneapolis: Future Systems Inc., 1980).

Gerald Weinberg, *An Introduction to General Systems Thinking* (New York: John Wiley & Sons, 1975).

Kevin Kelly, *Out of Control: The New Biology of Machines, Social Systems, and the Economic World* (New York: Addison-Wesley, 1994).

James Gleick, *Chaos: Making a New Science* (New York: Penguin Books, 1987).

Fritjof Capra, *The Turning Point: Science, Society, and the Rising Culture* (New York: Bantam Books, 1982).

Donald Wheeler, *Understanding Variation: The Key to Managing Chaos* (Knoxville TN: SPC Press, 1993).

10

Leadership and Values:
Creating an Organizational Culture

The modern health care organization, striving to succeed in an increasingly competitive environment, requires transformational leaders who can define shared values, articulate vitalizing visions, and develop innovative mental models. And the need is urgent. In Peter Senge's words:

> When all is said and done, learning organizations will remain a "good idea," an intriguing but distant vision until people take a stand for building such organizations. Taking this stand is the first leadership act, the start of inspiring (literally "to breathe life into") the vision of learning organizations. In the absence of this stand, the learning disciplines remain mere collections of tools and technique—means of solving problems rather than creating something genuinely new."[1]

But who are these new leaders? And what is their mission in the modern Knowledge Society? "One of the most universal cravings of our time," notes James MacGregor Burns, "is a hunger for creative leadership." But what is creative leadership? And, more specifically, what leadership style will best serve our complex health care organizations in a competitive and changing environment?

Traditional leadership models, deeply rooted in an individual-istic and nonsystemic worldview, have assumed over the years that followers lack vision and power—and the ability to master (or even understand) forces of change. In recent years, however, organizational theorists have moved toward a *systems* perspec-tive—toward the view that leaders and followers must *mutually co-produce* overall system leadership.

This new leadership philosophy—one that fits the learning or-ganization well—seeks to develop strong, committed, flexible, self-directed employees who find ways to improve continually their organization's processes and systems. And it rests on three bedrock concepts: *values, vision, and culture*. Before considering these concepts and their connection to leadership, let's look first at some differences between leadership and management.

Leaders and managers

Leaders often manage, and managers often lead—but their roles, functions, and tasks differ significantly. And, in the words of War-ren Bennis, "American organizations have been overmanaged and underled."

- *Managers* are appointed
  Leaders are chosen

- *Managers* master routines and increase efficiency.
  Leaders provide judgment and increase effectiveness.

- *Managers* plan, investigate, coordinate, evaluate,
    supervise, staff, negotiate, and represent.
  Leaders define basic purposes and point an
    organization in a general direction.

- *Managers* set targets or goals, establish detailed
    steps for achieving those goals, and allocate
    needed resources.

> *Leaders* develop a vision and formulate broad strategies for achieving that vision.

- *Managers* create processes that strive to implement plans precisely and efficiently.
  Leaders align people and move them in a desired direction.

- *Managers* use control mechanisms to determine congruency between system behavior and plan, and they take action to correct deviations.
  Leaders help individuals find achievement, recognition, self-esteem, a feeling of control, a sense of belonging, and the ability to live up to their ideals.

- *Managers* design effective processes and systems.
  Leaders articulate and institutionalize worthy ideals and values.

In his book *Mind of a Manager, Soul of a Leader*, Craig Hickman offers these distinctions:

The words *manager* and *leader* are metaphors representing two opposite ends of a continuum. *Manager* tends to signify the more analytical, structured, controlled, deliberate, and orderly end of the continuum, while *leader* tends to occupy the more experimental, visionary, flexible, uncontrolled, and creative end. Given these fairly universal metaphors of contrasting organizational behavior, I like to think of the prototypical manager as the person who brings the thoughts of the mind to bear on daily organizational problems. In contrast, the leader brings the feeling of the soul to bear on those same problems. Certainly, managers and leaders both have minds and souls, but they each tend to emphasize one over the other as they function in organizations. The mind represents the analytical, calculating, structuring, and ordering side of tasks and organizations. The soul, on the other hand, represents the visionary, passionate, creative, and flexible side.[2]

Our health care system needs major contributions from both managers *and* leaders. But it needs especially *transformational* leaders who can integrate the learning disciplines and foster an organizational culture that promotes change and renewal. *Transformational* leaders differ significantly from *transactional* leaders.

Transactional leaders excel at management functions. They strive to maintain a smooth, well-run operation and focus on tangible organizational elements—plans, schedules, budgets. They conform to organizational norms and almost always occupy administrative positions in the formal structure. And their leadership skills differ little from managers' skills.

Transformational leaders, on the other hand, influence and persuade—and embody the group's *values*. They inspire employees to raise performance levels, and they take calculated risks to stimulate change efforts. Tom Peters and Robert Waterman in their book *In Search of Excellence* define the transforming leader this way:

> The transforming leader is concerned with minutiae as well. But he is concerned with the tricks of the pedagogue, the mentor, the linguist—the more successfully to become the value-shaper, the exemplar, the maker of meanings. His job is much tougher than that of the transactional leader, for he is the true artist, the true pathfinder. After all, he is both calling forth and exemplifying the urge for transcendence that unites us all. At the same time, he exhibits almost boorish consistency over long periods of time in support of his one or two transcending values. No opportunity is too small, no forum too insignificant, no audience too junior.[3]

In addition to defining the transformational leader, Peters and Waterman also set forth in their 1982 book the intellectual outlines for a new leadership model—a new philosophy that rests on three broad values: 1) a concern for all organizational members, 2) an openness to change and innovation, and 3) a focus on quality service to employees and customers.

Although Peters and Waterman did not define the specific values that infuse the new leadership model, their discussion helped launch research into a values-driven, change-oriented, developmental *leadership philosophy* that fosters a common vision—and that creates and maintains a culture conducive to values-based decision-making. In the words of Gilbert Fairholm:

> The technology developing out of this philosophy of leadership is excellence in group action through empowerment. Leaders strengthen coworkers, teach them, and inspire them toward a common vision of what the group is and can become. The vision provides the group a values base for commitment. . . .These values also provide the basis for a unique excellence culture and new leadership skills. These skills are counciling with coworkers and teaching them values, vision aims, cultural mores, and excellence techniques so that they can govern themselves.[4]

Let's look more closely at the nature of modern leadership and it relation to the learning organization.

Leadership and the learning organization

Leaders are chosen. And followers expect leaders to embody the values and characteristics that promote organizational and individual success. Effective leaders demonstrate desired behaviors and attitudes—the essence of true leadership. But what kinds of characteristics elicit respect and admiration—and ultimately foster loyalty and followership? And what kinds of actions move organizational members in desired directions? Employees admire and respect specific actions:

> Actions that exemplify desired values and that foster congruence between individual and organizational values

> Actions that relate everyday activities to long-range organizational goals and vision

Actions that communicate the presence of predictability, honesty, and concern

Actions that indicate a concern in followers' interests as they relate to work, career, family, and extra-mural activities

Actions that indicate the leader's interest in self-knowledge and self-development

In all these actions, effective leaders treat coworkers and customers with the greatest respect and courtesy. And this respect manifests itself in a desire to provide the training and education that will promote personal development and individual success.

Employees look not only at leaders' actions but also at leaders' characteristics—their personal qualities. Leaders in the learning organization manifest their values through their behavior (they "walk the talk"), and they attract followers who share similar values. But certain mode of conduct values (or characteristics) seem more important than others. James Kouzes and Barry Posner, through a series of surveys, defined certain qualities that help leaders draw others into a common cause and commitment. The results of two surveys are shown in Table 2 (facing page).[5]

Respondent groups over a six-year period consistently rated four leadership characteristics highest. People want their leaders to be *honest*, *forward-looking*, *inspiring*, and *competent*. And the results of the two surveys differ only slightly, indicating that the most admired qualities and the overall mode of conduct value hierarchies remained remarkably stable over time.

A leader's values, characteristics, and actions all contribute to the creation and development of an organizational culture. But what is organizational culture? And what's its relation to *excellence* and *stakeholder development*—the two central guiding principles of values leadership?

TABLE 2

Characteristics of Admired Leaders

Characteristic	1993 U.S. Respondents Percentage of People Selecting	1987 U.S. Respondents Percentage of People Selecting
Honest	87	83
Forward-looking	71	62
Inspiring	68	58
Competent	58	67
Fair-minded	49	40
Supportive	46	32
Broad-minded	41	37
Intelligent	38	43
Straightforward	34	34
Courageous	33	27
Dependable	32	32
Cooperative	30	25
Imaginative	28	34
Caring	27	26
Mature	14	23
Determined	13	20
Ambitious	10	21
Loyal	10	11
Self-controlled	5	13
Independent	5	10

Leadership and culture

All organizations possess a distinct culture. And visitors to an organization (including customers and potential employees) can quickly perceive or "feel" the nature of the culture. But what nourishes and sustains a desired culture—and keeps it open to change and innovation?

The term *culture* has been defined in various ways over the years, and social scientists and other theorists continue to debate the nature and function of organizational culture. Marshall Sashkin and Kenneth Kiser in their book *Putting Total Quality Management to Work* define organizational culture as:

... the cumulative perception of how the organization treats people and how people expect to treat one another. It is based on consistent and persistent management action, as seen by employees, vendors, and customers.[6]

Organizational culture, say Sashkin and Kiser, derives from (perhaps consists of) certain fundamental beliefs and values. And the most difficult part of TQM to understand is the most important part: *creating, nurturing, and sustaining a TQM culture.*

Edgar Schein, an organizational theorist, defines the culture of a group as:

... the pattern of shared basic assumptions that the group learned as it solved its problems of external adaptation and internal integration, that has worked well enough to be considered valid and, therefore, to be taught to new members as the correct way to perceive, think, and feel in relation to those problems.[7]

We can, says Schein, analyze an organization in terms of its *norms, values, behavior patterns, rituals, and traditions.* But the culture concept adds two critical elements to the "sharing concept."

First, culture implies some level of *structural stability* in the group—a deep, shared experience and set of shared values that provide stability and meaning. Second, culture somehow implies that the organizational rituals, climate, values, and behaviors bind together into a coherent whole—into patterns that eventually reveal themselves as "culture." Cultural formation is thus, by definition, always a striving toward *patterning and integration*— even though the history and experience of most groups prevents them from ever achieving a fully clear-cut paradigm.[8]

All leadership actions contribute in some way (for better or worse) to the creation, maintenance, and transformation of organizational culture. Effective leaders, however, strive to institute *planned* programs of culture development and management— a three-step process:

- *First*, working with key stakeholders, they establish explicit goals and norms and then attempt to identify hidden goals and balancing loops that may be over-riding and subverting the organization's stated goals. And they attempt to answer the question, "What's re-ally driving the organization, and are those forces in-congruent with expressed goals?"
- *Second*, they identify the cultural values, norms, and behaviors that will move the organization in desired directions.
- *Third*, they formally articulate the norms and values that will foster a culture dedicated to productive change.

Organizations develop cultures that reflect the values and practices of their leaders. Learning organization leaders use various strategies to develop their cultures, but three activities seem critical to an effective values leadership style—*modeling, teaching, and counciling*. And these *transformational* leadership activities represent a departure from traditional *transactional* leadership behaviors.

Modeling

Leaders communicate their values and preferences in various ways, but effective values leaders first and foremost *model* desired behaviors. That is, they display attitudes—and consciously engage in actions—that convey their expectations. These actions and attitudes include, for example:

- *Respectful treatment of others (common courtesy)*
- *Face-to-face contact with a wide variety of stakehold-ers (management by wandering around)*
- *Frequent association with stakeholders in joint plan-ning and decision-making (caring and counciling)*

- *Conscious actions that reinforce the organizations vision (strategic vision focus)*
- *Listening in a way that communicates genuine interest and optimizes understanding (focused listening)*
- *Use of symbols that recognize shared values and reinforce the core-vision value (symbol use)*
- *Group gatherings that recognize and honor individual performance (celebrations)*

Leaders who model desired behaviors present a picture of the "collective mental model" they wish to foster. And no modeling activity is more critical than the leader's demonstrated interest in *his or her* own education and self-development. In the learning organization, education and knowledge provide the fuel that sparks new understandings, new ideas, and new challenges. And effective leaders in the new learning organization discover not just how to learn but how to learn *in an organizational context*—and how to motivate others to learn and develop.

Values leaders stimulate learning by demonstrating an ongoing commitment to both "maintenance" and "innovative" learning. The Club of Rome (an ad hoc group) makes this distinction:

> Maintenance learning is the acquisition of fixed outlooks, methods, and rules for dealing with known and recurring situations. It enhances our problem-solving ability for problems that are given. It is the type of learning designed to maintain an existing system or an established way of life. Maintenance learning is, and will continue to be, indispensable to the functioning and stability of every society. But for long-term survival, particularly in times of turbulence, change, or discontinuity, another type of learning is even more essential. It is the type of learning that can bring change, renewal, restructuring, and problem reformulation—and which we have called innovative learning.[9]

Maintenance learning tends to focus on knowledge required to maintain an existing system, and many managers gravitate toward maintenance learning. Innovative learning, however, addresses *emerging* issues—problems and opportunities that lack precedent and that require new contexts. Learning organization leaders must continue to model admired characteristics—honesty, competency, fair-mindedness, dependability, and courage, for example. But they will advance their organization's culture and productivity by presenting an innovative learning model that helps organizational members anticipate and respond to changing circumstances—and helps them reliably predict the future.

Teaching

Leaders also teach, and the true values leader understands the essence of inspirational leadership—the *psychological* and *educational* development of others. Leadership can be viewed as a teaching activity that creates a learning environment and that strives to develop skills, self-governance, and effectiveness. Learning organization leaders empower employees by clarifying the path to organizational and individual success and reducing or eliminating the roadblocks and pitfalls along the way. They take into account the personal characteristics of their followers (abilities, skills, needs, interests, motivations) and the environmental variables that influence followers. And they help all employees develop the ability to govern their work lives, further their career interests, enhance their extra-mural lives—and ultimately achieve personal, professional, and organizational goals.

In so doing, they create still more leaders—leaders imbued with similar core values and ideals and dedicated to helping the organization attain its vision. Leaders meld other leaders into a unified system focused on common goals and bound by shared values.

Values leaders (teachers all) form a relationship of trust with their followers and establish an ethic of service. They think in terms of *value systems* rather than *control systems*, and they form a collegial and sharing relationship with their followers. They sit in council with them, formulating and initiating joint actions—and using *dialogue* to promote mutually acceptable visions, strategies, and goals.

Counciling

Modern leaders "sit in council" with their followers, engaging in one-on-one exchanges that seek to develop a common culture, vision, and set of values—and a common understanding of work processes and goals. Counciling activities recognize employees' feelings. They stress passion, emotion, and commitment. And they strive always to promote simultaneously the interests of the stakeholders *and* the organization.

The counciling model seeks to move away from traditional leadership models that have viewed employees as tools for helping leaders and managers achieve their goals. Counciling moves leaders into a more personal, intimate, face-to-face transaction that puts the leader and follower on an equal footing—and that helps both discover the right, proper, and needed directions.

Leadership and values

Leaders deal in norms, attitudes, and motivations. But the modern leader in the new learning organization understands that *values* shape organizational norms and structure—and that effective leaders work incessantly to establish, clarify, communicate, and guard organizational values. Values leaders help the organization integrate and energize its multidimensionally talented members. And they help develop both an organization's end-state of existence values (its ultimate objectives) and its mode of conduct values (the behaviors that advance the organization toward its objectives). Leaders who define and articulate shared values—and then integrate them into the organization—foster an organizational culture that helps stakeholders (often a highly diverse lot) find congruence between their values and the organization's values.

Diversity needn't splinter organizational life and culture. Indeed, diversity represents both an opportunity and a challenge. John Gardner puts it this way:

> [Your goal is] not to achieve wholeness by suppressing diversity, nor to make wholeness impossible by enthroning diversity, but to preserve both. Each element in the diversity must be respected, but each must ask itself sincerely what it can contribute to the whole. I don't think it is venturing beyond the truth to say that "wholeness incorporating diversity" defines the transcendent task for our generation.[10]

The new values leadership philosophy, then, takes into account diversity and individuality and seeks "wholeness incorporating diversity." But it also assumes a culture of excellence and general agreement about the value context in which all organizational members will operate. Without such agreement, employees may tend to follow their individual interests—and to develop activities that subvert cooperative action and organizational goals. A set of shared values, however, will ultimately promote the development and attainment of a shared organizational *vision* that mobilizes energies and inspires joint actions.

Leadership and vision

Leaders set and articulate the organization's vitalizing vision, an activity that helps organizational members implement values and purposes. A vision integrates values—and unifies and coordinates employees' actions around central values. *And a shared vision constitutes one of the most powerful forces in organizational life.*

A shared vision creates a common identity and binds organizational members together in common goals and aspirations. It focuses and energizes employees. And it projects a realistic, credible, and promising future for the organization. A shared vision helps an organization define a clear purpose and helps individuals find their organizational roles. In the words of Peter Senge:

> You cannot have a learning organization without a shared vision. Without a pull toward some goal which people truly want to achieve, the forces in support of the status quo can be overwhelming. Vision establishes an overarching goal. The loftiness of the target compels new ways of thinking and acting. A shared vision also provides a rudder to keep the learning process on course when stresses develop. Learning can be difficult, even painful. With a shared vision, we are more likely to expose our ways of thinking, give up deeply-held views, and recognize personal and organizational shortcomings.[11]

With all the benefits a vision provides, why don't leaders simply "install" a vision worthy of commitment—and be done with it? Visions occasionally emanate from the top, but only rarely do they take root through edict. More often visions "bubble up" through various levels in the organization. The values leader helps identify the vision, articulate it, and express the image or metaphor that makes it "feel right"—that helps all the actors buy into it. A leader who can sort through all the images, signals, forecasts, and alternatives that an organization produces—and then synthesize and assemble a vision—possesses a transcending ability to set daily events into a larger context.

The effective leader, however, also must take the next step: he or she must possess the ability to *communicate* the vision throughout the entire organization. In the words of Bert Nanus:

> Leaders are only as powerful as the ideas they can communicate. The leader's basic philosophy must be: 'We have seen what this organization can be, we understand the consequences of that vision, and now we must act to make it so.'[12]

Visionary, values leaders seek answers to broad-gauged questions. What is our role or service—our "business?" Who are our clients and customers? Our competitors? What are the forces that are driving change in the organization, the community, and the broad social environment? What are the technological, social, and intellectual ideas that may shape the organization's future? Visionary leaders select, organize, structure, and interpret information that helps them predict the future and construct not only a *vision* but also a *strategic plan*. Out of the strategic plan come short-range and mid-range goals that are consistent with the organization's vision.

Effective values leadership, however, requires far more than the ability to articulate shared values and to set forth a clear, shared vision. It also requires the ability to harmonize complexity and mediate dilemmas— and the willingness and ability to exercise *power*. And the relation between leadership and power is one of the least understood elements in leadership theory.

Leadership and power

Power, the *potential* for one individual or group to influence the behavior of another individual or group, often determines who gets what—and when and how. Powerholders daily shape (often dominate) organizational affairs. Yet, we understand little about the nature of power and its relation to organizational change. And we understand even less about the ways leaders can use their sources of power to achieve productive ends. Warren Bennis and Burt Nanus, in their discussion of various leadership models, note:

> . . . there is something missing from all the "new age" formulations—one issue which has been systematically neglected without exception: *power, the basic energy to initiate and sustain action translating intention into reality*, the quality without which leaders cannot lead. Just as the economists have painted themselves

into a narrowing corner by failing to recognize the limitations and constraints of the free market, so too have students of organizations avoided the nucleus of leadership. Without any qualification, we can bluntly state that all of the current paradigms of organizational life, be they the 'new age' variety or the older brands, have failed to consider *power*.[13]

In American society, the term *power* is loaded with negative connotations, and individuals who seek power often acquire the pejorative label *power hungry*. But power is a means and not an end. As such, it can be used for rational, benevolent, and inspiring purposes—as well as for irrational, malicious, and self-interested ends. Leaders who understand the full range of their power sources dramatically increase their leadership potential.

Sources of power

To initiate and implement innovations, organizational leaders and "change agents" need the power to disrupt "business as usual"—to move the system off course and sail it into uncharted seas. But leaders cannot just simply command their colleagues and co-workers. Neither can they ignore their critics. They must understand their *legitimate sources of power*, and they must acquire the political skills that will help them translate power into action. But what are these sources of power? And how can values leaders tap into them?

The work of French and Raven is often cited in discussions about power. Building on their work, Hersey, Blanchard, and Natemeyer have defined eight sources of leadership power.[14]

> · *Coercive power* is based on the perception that an individual has the authority to punish or recommend punishment. Its base is fear and the power to criticize, demote, fire, reprimand, and influence financial compensations.

- *Reward power* (or persuasive power) is based on the perception that an individual can provide important formal rewards such as pay increases and promotions or more subjective rewards such as praise, attention, recognition, and opportunities for self-development.
- *Legitimate power* is based on the possession of certain licenses or credentials—or on the perception that an individual possesses the ability to influence others through his or her formal position or role.
- *Referent power* (or charismatic power) is based on the ability to elicit respect, admiration, emulation—and a desire for association.
- *Knowledge power* (or expert power) is based on the perception that an individual possesses the skill, knowledge, expertise, and judgment to help an organization or individual achieve certain objectives.
- *Information power* is based on the perception that an individual possesses (or has access to) valuable information that can promote another's interests.
- *Resource power* (often related to position power) is based on the perception that an individual possesses the ability to control a critical, scarce, or nonsubstitutable resources essential to the organization's well-being.
- *Access power* (or connection power) is based on the perception that an individual possesses access to powerful individuals or groups or to other forms of power.

Effective leaders recognize the source (or sources) of power that will best serve them in a given context or set of circumstances. And they call on all their available power sources. In our new Knowledge Society, however (a society that rests on "knowledge work" and "knowledge workers"), effective leaders rely heavily on *knowledge-based power*—on the ability to ask the right questions and to analyze the data in ways that help predict the future. Since today's basic economic resource is now knowledge, effective leaders will need to allocate knowledge as productively as earlier leaders allocated capital and materials.

Competence—the application of knowledge and expertise and the exercise of good judgement—also appeals to many organizational members, and its use tends to increase satisfaction and performance levels. Competence may be viewed as the ability 1) to predict the future, 2) to recognize opportunities, and 3) to maintain efficiency and effectiveness. Incompetent leaders quickly lose their followers—and may adopt coercive measures to maintain their influence.

Reward power is often associated with the ability to provide financial or other material rewards, but some analysts question the efficacy of those rewards. Reward power becomes a real force when it is used to recognize the intrinsic worth of individuals and to help them grow and succeed.

Most organizational members reject *coercive* power. Coercive power (the "big stick" approach) imposes a psychological and emotional burden on both leaders *and* followers. It encourages suspicion, deceit, and dishonesty—and it exerts a reactive and temporary influence. It dissipates quickly when the coercive leader or controlling system disappears.

Again, effective leaders make full use of their various power sources, and they learn to use the source that will best serve them in a specific setting or context. Often, however, leaders who lack *coercive* power readily conclude that they lack *all* sources of power—and they abdicate their leadership role. They fail to recognize (and implement) the many other power sources available to them. Few leaders possess access to all forms of power. But leaders who understand their many power sources (and the limitations of coercive power) will optimize and strengthen their leadership role over time—and ultimately enhance their influence. Such leaders will not only endure, they will prevail.

Getting past no

We identify shared values (and find common agreement) through a *process* that seeks to include the perspectives of all organizational members. A fair process helps *all* employees participate in the quest to find common purpose and a community of shared values. And effective leaders will ensure that all employees have the opportunity to address basic questions. What values do we hold deeply? And do they make any difference? Good leaders help their constituents avoid asking, What values *should* we hold?—a question that leads only to empty rhetorical statements and justifiable cynicism.

Leaders and other employees frequently hit roadblocks in their attempts to align individual and organizational values. And they often blame stalemates on "the others." Harvard Professor William Ury in his book *Getting Past No* notes that leaders can help employees build a "golden bridge" to agreement. This golden bridge helps people overcome four common obstacles to reaching consensus: 1) it's not my idea, 2) it doesn't meet my needs, 3) it may embarrass me, and 4) it asks me to do too much too quickly.[15]

Ury provides some basic advice to organizational members attempting to relieve values conflicts: resist pushing your own ideas and values, he says, and establish a *process* for involving all others in the conflict resolution. Resolution sometimes comes about through identifying a higher order value and a new interdependency. But the process for reconciling value dilemmas and finding shared values is not without risks. In the words of Charles Hampden-Turner, a senior research fellow at the London School of Business:

Confronting dilemmas is both dangerous and potentially reward-ing. Opposing values 'crucify' the psyche and threaten to dis-integrate both leader and organization. Yet to resolve these same tensions enables the organization to create wealth and outper-form competitors. If you duck the dilemma you also miss the res-olution. There is no cheap grace.[16]

Conclusion

Values leadership possesses two critical and overarching di-mensions that distinguish it from all the other leadership con-cepts. First, it strives always toward *excellence*—the standard for individual and collective performance among all stakehold-ers. Second, it emphasizes above all the concept of *stakehold-er development*—the fullest development of all organizational members and the development of independent, self-directing teams that relentlessly pursue excellence and continuous quality improvement.

Most leadership theories espouse excellence and personal de-velopment to some degree or another. The new values leadership approach differs, however, in its unflinching insistence on individ-ual growth and development—an emphasis that represents a radi-cal shift in both leadership thinking and leader behavior. And the modern leadership values philosophy—a system of principles, val-ues, and perspectives—holds great potential for steering leaders toward interactions that mutually co-produce leadership and truly transform organizational culture.

REFERENCES

1. Peter Senge, *The Fifth Discipline: The Art & Practice of the Learning Organization* (New York: Doubleday, 1990), 340.
2. Craig Hickman, *Mind of a Manager, Soul of a Leader* (New York: John Wiley & Sons, 1990), 7.
3. Thomas Peters and Robert Waterman, *In Search of Excellence* (New York: Warner Books, 1984), 82–83.
4. Gilbert Fairholm, *Values Leadership: Toward a New Philosophy of Leadership* (Westport CT: Praeger Publishers, 1991).
5. James Kouzes and Barry Posner, *The Leadership Challenge: How to Get Extraordinary Things Done in Organizations* (San Francisco: Jossey-Bass, 1987).
6. Marshall Sashkin and Kenneth Kiser, *Putting Total Quality Management to Work* (San Francisco: Berrett-Koehler, 1993), 111.
7. Edgar Schein, *Organizational Culture and Leadership* (San Francisco: Jossey-Bass, 1992), 315.
8. Ibid., 315.
9. James Botkin, Elmandjra Mahdi, and Malitza Mircea, *No Limits to Learning* (New York: Pergamon Press), 10.
10. John Gardner, *Building Community* (Washington D.C.: Independent Sector, 1991).
11. Senge, *The Fifth Discipline*, 209.
12. Burt Nanus, *Visionary Leadership* (San Francisco: Jossey-Bass, 1992).
13. Warren Bennis and Burt Nanus, *Leaders: The Strategies for Taking Charge* (New York: Harper & Row, 1985), 15.
14. Paul Hersey and Kenneth Blanchard, *Management of Organizational Behavior* (Englewood Cliffs NJ: Prentice-Hall, 1982).
15. William Ury, *Getting to Yes: Negotiating Agreement Without Giving In* (New York: Penguin Books, 1983).
16. Charles Hampden-Turner, *Creating Corporate Culture: From Discord to Harmony* (New York: Addison-Wesley, 1990).

SUGGESTED READINGS

J. Thomas Wren, ed., *The Leader's Companion: Insights on Leadership Through the Ages* (New York: Free Press, 1995).
Burt Nanus, *Visionary Leadership* (San Francisco: Jossey-Bass, 1992).
Margaret Wheatley, *Leadership and the New Science* (San Francisco: Berrett-Koehler, 1992).
Gilbert Fairholm, *Values Leadership: Toward a New Philosophy of Leadership* (Westport CT: Praeger Publishers, 1991).
B. M. Bass, *Bass and Stodgill's Handbook of Leadership* (New York: Free Press, 1990).

11

Medical Education:
Broadening the Perspective

Educators and other analysts have long decried the state of American medical education. In his 1879 annual report, Harvard College president Charles Eliot observed: "The ignorance and general incompetency of the average graduate of American Medical Schools, at the time when he receives the degree which turns him loose upon the community, is something horrible to contemplate." The next year Eliot came directly to the point: "The whole system of medical education in this country" he said, "needs thorough reformation."[1]

As we approach the twenty-first century, calls for medical education reform continue. In a report entitled *Medical Education in Transition*, the Robert Wood Johnson Foundation Commission on Medical Education noted that five national commissions over the past fifteen years have called for greater congruence between academic medicine's activities and the public's changing health care expectations.[2]

Despite the insistent calls for reform (greater now, perhaps, than at any time since the turn of the century), medical education—influenced by vested bureaucratic and financial interests—continues to stay socially organized and structured in ways that inhibit change and innovation. And important sectors in American society (public and private) continue to question medical education's interest in the major health care issues of the day. Today's medical educators face large questions:

- What is academic medicine's role in identifying and addressing broad social health care issues?
- What kinds of physicians (and how many) will help society meet its growing health care needs?
- What new teaching and scholarship approaches will help academic medical centers meet modern health care challenges?

Before addressing these and other questions, let's look first at the growing discontinuity between American medical education and society's broad health care expectations.

Academic medicine and the social contract

American academic medicine operates under an unwritten *social contract* with the American public. This unstated social covenant— a broad, implicit agreement that defines certain rights and duties— rests on the premise that the medical academy's programs and commitments will 1) provide scientifically trained physicians and other health care workers, 2) will conduct biomedical research activities that address disease processes, and 3) will continue to focus on *individual* care needs—while also addressing certain *social* health care issues.

Over the past fifty years, the medical social contract has served us well. The public has endowed the medical profession with influence, resources, status, and autonomy. And, in turn, the medical profession, led by its medical school faculties, has identified and helped ameliorate critical individual and collective health problems. The medical education enterprise has trained a superb corps of scientists, physicians, and other health care professionals who have developed the world's most sophisticated set of patient care services—and who continue to make stunning contributions.

Yet, despite academic medicine's incomparable successes, the public senses a growing discontinuity between medical education's focus and society's changing (and growing) health care needs. And, as we move toward the next century, we hear increasing demands for a more balanced set of health goals and objectives and a greater recognition 1) that health and health care lie imbedded in a *social context* and 2) that educators, practitioners, and policy makers must find more ways to integrate the *population perspective* into their traditional *patient-centered* and *biotechnical* strategies. But how can we begin to bring these broad population and social perspectives into focus?

Leonard Duhl sees two related but distinct approaches to the study of social environmental influences on health. In his words:

> The first uses statistical and epidemiological techniques to correlate such factors as education, race, economic status, age, and occupation with the incidence of illness and injury. The second, a more broadly cultural approach to the relationship between social environment and health, considers the influence of 'softer' factors on health and illness. Among its concerns are the structure of social networks, the influence of the mass media on people's attitudes and beliefs, the freedom or lack of it to grow and develop normally and naturally, the effects of community politics and participation, the ways in which social settings foster or frustrate self-esteem and confidence. Although the second approach makes use of some of the statistical information provided by the first, it tends to avoid statistical analysis and must be defined in more intuitive, speculative ways. Both approaches, applied together, can help health planners and policy makers—and, indeed, individual practitioners—take action to affect the health of groups within their scope.[3]

Professor Duhl's appeal for a two-pronged approach to the analysis of environmental health influences reminds us of the complexities surrounding health and health care—and the urgent need for medicine 1) to promote healthy family and community environments and 2) to address the social pathologies that undermine health and ultimately burden the care system. "Let the health care system continue as it is," argues Duhl, " but let us narrow its responsibilities." And if we can lighten its load, he says, we might "find ways to finance what it can do best."

Many medical educators and health policy analysts support the public's increasing demand for broader and more holistic approaches to health care—and, yet, professional schools continue to resist the *population perspective*. For various complex (often legitimate), reasons, they hold closely to the medical "cure and care" model. And the gap between academic medical goals and broad social goals continues to widen. Where then do we go? How do we begin developing greater congruence between academic medical activities and the public's unmet health care needs? And who will lead the way?

Medical education and the academic physician

All physicians can find ways to further medical education efforts. But academic physicians are uniquely positioned to move the medical enterprise forward. It is they who select the physicians of the future. It is they who supervise medical education. And it is they who significantly shape the values, beliefs, attitudes, perspectives, interests, and priorities of future physicians—including future academic physicians.

Academic medical specialists determine research agendas, provide leadership for professional schools and associations, and (more often than not) control virtually all the points at which critical professional decisions are made. Decisions by representatives of medical schools, teaching hospitals, specialty associations, and credentialing bodies drive the medical profession's collective response to the public's health issues. And, increasingly, the public is looking to medical centers and their faculties for guidance on social health policy issues. But how should American academic medicine respond to the nation's social health needs? Can the academy redefine its role and reshape its activities in ways that will meet tomorrow's challenges? And can it redefine and strengthen its long-standing social contract with the American public?

Change and innovation in medical academic centers occurs slowly. Major "externalities" (government financing mechanisms, for example) powerfully influence decision making within the academic medical center—and often inhibit educational reform. Moreover, proposed changes in medical school curriculums are critically reviewed by a variety of bodies, including accrediting organizations, semiautonomous departments within the school, affiliated hospitals, professional organizations within the medical community, and financing authorities. And various power interests frequently conflict in ways that impede change efforts.

Despite daunting obstacles to change, academic medicine's role in reform activities remains critical *And the academy must look both to its internal and external environments.* That is, while developing new approaches to scholarship and teaching, the medical academy must also strengthen its contribution to the common social good. And faculties (including administrators) seeking to redefine academic roles and cultures might begin by examining their view of *scholarship*.

Scholarship: enlarging the perspective

Medical school faculties face a complex future. They must continue to fulfill traditional expectations—while setting forth visions that will help medical professionals meet the changing requirements of a complex health care world. And their success in reformulating roles and relationship—and meeting diverse expectations—will rest heavily on their ability to develop (and then reward) a more inclusive view of *scholarship*.

In *Scholarship Reconsidered*, a report published by the Carnegie Foundation for the Advancement of Teaching, the late Ernest Boyer urged educators to clarify campus missions and reconsider the meaning of scholarship.[4] His observations, directed toward all higher education institutions, merit the attention of medical educators seeking a less restrictive view of scholarship and a reconsideration of the professoriate's priorities. And we are indebted to professor Boyer for his keen analysis and penetrating insights.

Scholarship revisited

Scholarship in American higher education has moved through three distinct (but overlapping) phases. The colonial college, influenced by its British heritage, focused on "character building" and preparation for civic and religious leadership. And its faculty, hewing to certain religious dictates, mainly promoted intellectual, moral, and spiritual development. In the words of historian Theodore Benditt: "Professors were hired not for their scholarly ability or achievement but for their religious commitment. Scholarly achievement was not a high priority."[5]

This emphasis on teaching persisted well into the nineteenth century, when nation building and the requirements of industrial capitalism gave rise to the Land Grant College Act and the idea of *service*. And both private and public colleges and universities met the challenge. In 1903, David Starr Jordan, president of Stanford University, declared that the entire twentieth-century university movement "is toward reality and practicality."[6] And in 1908, Harvard president Charles Eliot claimed: "At bottom most of the American institutions of higher education are filled with the modern democratic spirit of serviceableness. Teachers and students alike are profoundly moved by the desire to serve the democratic community. . . . All the colleges boast of the serviceable men they have trained, and regard the serviceable patriot as their ideal product. This is a thoroughly democratic conception of their function."[7]

In the late nineteenth century, the advancement of knowledge through *research* had taken firm root in American higher education. And throughout the first half of the twentieth century, the emphasis on teaching and service steadily lost ground—even as (paradoxically) higher education's mission had expanded to become (in the words of a 1947 presidential commission report) "the means by which every citizen, youth, and adult, is enabled and encouraged to carry his education, formal and informal, as far as his native capacities permit."

But even as higher education's mission expanded throughout the 1940s and 1950s, the standards for evaluating professorial achievement and academic prestige increasingly focused on research and published results. And in just a few decades, the research element of scholarship had gained preeminence. Although the modern academy regularly declares undying support for teaching and service activities, research programs continue to dominate—and promotions and rewards go heavily in *research* directions.

Against this brief historical backdrop, some central questions present themselves. Can academic medical centers broaden and redefine the rigid teaching, service, and research categories—and then redefine the meaning of scholarship? Can they move beyond the tired old "teaching versus research" debate? Can they broaden the scope of academic work and find more effective ways to evaluate and reward teaching skills? And can they define faculty activities in ways that more realistically reflect academic and civic mandates?

We think the answer to all these questions is "yes." But first academicians need to consider the full range of scholarship—and the interrelations between and among four specific, yet overlapping, scholarly functions: the scholarship of *discovery*, the scholarship of *integration*, the scholarship of *application*, and the scholarship of *teaching*. Let's look briefly at each.

Discovery

The scholarship of discovery—the element in the model that most closely resembles traditional academic "research"—reflects, in William Bowen's words, "our pressing, irrepressible need as human beings to confront the unknown and to seek understanding for its own sake." This search, says Bowen, "is tied inextricably to the freedom to think freshly, to see propositions of every kind in ever-changing light—and it celebrates the special exhilaration that comes from a new idea."[8]

Scholarly investigation lies at the heart of academic life, and few academicians (if any) challenge its value—although they continue to question its prominence. Discovery contributes not only to the store of human knowledge but also to the intellectual climate of colleges and universities. The researcher's probing pursuit of knowledge invigorates and enlivens the academy—and ultimately nourishes all our institutions. And the pursuit of knowledge must be assiduously cultivated and defended. But today's complex world requires more than discovery; it also demands *integration*.

Integration

The *scholarship of integration* requires the ability to make connections across the disciplines, to place the specialties in a larger context, and then to illuminate data in a revealing way. Integration puts isolated facts in perspective and gives them meaning, and it trains fresh insights on original research. Mark Van Doren gave expression to this integrated view of knowledge when he observed:

> The connectedness of things is what the educator contemplates to the limit of his capacity. No human capacity is great enough to permit a vision of the world as simple, but if the educator does not aim at the vision no one else will, and the consequences are dire when no one does.[9]

The scholarship of integration, closely related to the scholarship of discovery, involves research at the boundaries where disciplines converge and academic neighborhoods overlap. But integration also asks scholars to fit their research findings (or others' findings) into larger intellectual patterns—and then to interpret those patterns. Discovery scholars must continue to ask their central questions (What is yet to be known? What is yet to be found?). But integration scholars must ask other questions (What do the findings *mean*? And can we interpret our discoveries in ways that provide larger, more comprehensive understandings?).

Integrative scholarly activity requires critical analytic and interpretive skills—and the ability to move beyond the boundaries of traditional academic disciplines. In the words of Clifford Geertz, these shifts represent a fundamental "refiguration, . . . a phenomenon general enough to suggest that what we are seeing is not just another redrawing of the cultural map—the moving of a few disputed borders, the marking of some more picturesque mountain lakes—but an alteration of the principles of mapping."

"Something is happening," says Geertz, "to the way we think about the way we think." We are learning to think integratively, and integrative thinking can lead us from information to knowledge—perhaps even to wisdom. Moreover, the scholarship of *discovery* and *integration* can lead scholars to a third kind of activity—the scholarship of *application*.[10]

Application

The scholarship of discovery and the integration of knowledge reflect the investigative and synthesizing traditions of academic life, and they move us toward the *application* of knowledge—and still more questions. How can knowledge be responsibly applied to consequential problems? How can it be helpful to individuals as well as institutions? Can social problems themselves define an agenda for scholarly investigation?

One observer notes that scholarship has been defined by the British as "a means and measure of self-development," by the Germans as "an end in itself," and by Americans as "*equipment for service.*" The term *service*, however, eludes precise definition. And colleges and universities have tended to put distance between service activities (often tied to citizenship activities) and serious intellectual pursuits. But some service activities, especially those tied to a special field of knowledge, relate directly to professional endeavors. And certain kinds of serious and demanding service require the rigor and accountability we usually associate with research activities. Jencks and Reisman note that when free-standing professional schools affiliate with universities, they lessen their commitment to applied work. Professional schools associated with universities have fostered, in their words, "a more academic and less practical view of what their students need to know."[11]

The scholarship of *application*, then, goes beyond the view that knowledge is first "discovered" and then "applied." The process is more dynamic. In the act of application, theory and practice interact—and one renews the other. And scholarly service holds the potential for both *contributing* to human knowledge—and *applying* it to complex problems. In the words of Oscar Handlin, our troubled planet "can no longer afford the luxury of pursuits confined to an ivory tower. . . . [And] scholarship has to prove its worth not on its own terms but by service to the nation and the world."[12]

Teaching

Finally, the scholarship of *teaching*. Teaching, the highest form of understanding, creates a common ground of intellectual commitment. Good teachers stimulate active learning and foster critical, creative thinkers. And teaching not only *transmits* knowledge—it *transforms* and *extends* it. Inspired teaching keeps alive the flame of scholarship and maintains the continuity of knowledge. Physicist Robert Oppenheimer notes:

> The specialization of science is an inevitable accompaniment of progress; yet it is full of dangers, and it is cruelly wasteful, since so much that is beautiful and enlightening is cut off from most of the world. Thus it is proper to the role of the scientist that he not merely find the truth and communicate it to his fellows, but that he teach, that he try to bring the most honest and most intelligible account of new knowledge to all who will try to learn.[12]

All colleges and universities affirm the value of good teaching. But we've yet to redefine academic reward systems in ways that fully support and advance the teaching function—and that check the consuming preoccupation with research and publishing activities. Christopher Jenks and David Reisman note:

> No doubt most professors prefer it when their courses are popular, their lectures applauded, and their former students appreciative. But since such successes are of no help in getting a salary increase, moving to a more prestigious campus, or winning their colleagues' admiration, they are unlikely to struggle as hard to create them as to do other things. . . . Many potentially competent teachers do a conspicuously bad job in the classroom because they know that bad teaching is not penalized in any formal way.[13]

What then do we conclude? How can a more inclusive view of scholarship—a full appreciation of the discovery, integration, application, and teaching functions—advance academic medicine's mission?

First, a fuller recognition of all functions (and a redefined reward system) might allow a more flexible and varied approach to academic activities. At various points (depending on interests and opportunities), faculty members might wish to pursue specialized research, or to examine integrative questions, or to write interpretive articles—or to focus on specific application or teaching projects. Lee Knefelkamp of Columbia University has urged that academic life be seen through a "seasons" metaphor—and that faculty members be given the opportunity to change their interests and "revisit tasks, challenges, phases, stages—seasons—dozens of times during academic careers. There is no rhythm that fits every person. . . ."[14]

Moreover, a broader and richer view of scholarship might move faculty members toward a shared *vision* of intellectual and social possibilities—toward collaborative teaching and cooperative research activities that unite a "community of scholars" and strengthen its links to the broad society. Derek Bok, former Harvard president has noted the danger of further detachment:

> Armed with the security of tenure and the time to study the world with care, professors would appear to have a unique opportunity to act as society's scouts to signal impending problems long before they are visible to others. Yet rarely have members of the academy succeeded in discovering the emerging issues and bringing them vividly to the attention of the public.[15]

Learning activities are finally communal acts, and all stakeholders (students, teachers, and administrators) mutually enrich themselves when they honor good teaching and strive to bring teaching and research functions into better balance. Yet, prospective college teachers rarely bother to explore established educational concepts and proven teaching strategies. And even experienced teachers overlook the diverse nature of today's learners—many of whom bring adult experiences into the educational setting.

Malcolm Knowles has identified some adult learner characteristics. And his observations—together with Benjamin Bloom's analysis of various learning levels—illustrate some of the complexities surrounding today's teaching endeavor. Their formulations also indicate 1) the kinds of knowledge that can foster new teaching and learning approaches and 2) the types of concepts that can support a new educational model.

Characteristics of adult learners

Adult learners possess some special characteristics:

- They prefer learning experiences that meet their needs and interests.
- They prefer learning experiences that relate to their life experiences and circumstances.
- They prefer learning experiences that allow them to gather the most relevant and reliable information.
- They prefer learning experiences that involve a process of mutual inquiry.
- They prefer learning experiences that consider individual variations in learning style and pace.[16]

The exponential growth of medical knowledge has far exceeded individuals' capacity to store medical "facts." And, indeed, medicine's accelerating (almost dizzying) pace of change requires more than the ability to "pack facts." It demands the ability to understand principles and develop fact retrieval skills. And it requires *inner-directed, self-operating, life-long* learners who can effectively and creatively gather, analyze, integrate, synthesize, and evaluate information over their entire career span.

Some knowledge of adult learner characteristics may help students and teachers develop the life-long learning skills that will meet today's (and tomorrow's) professional challenges. And some introduction to the *levels of learning* concept may help both students and teachers increase their efficiency and effectiveness.

Levels of learning

In his noted work *Taxonomy of Educational Objectives, Handbook 1: Cognitive Domain*, Benjamin Bloom describes six major levels of learning: *knowledge, comprehension, application, analysis, synthesis, and evaluation.*[17] Learning, in Bloom's view, occurs at all these levels. But when self-directed learners and student-centered teachers mutually determine educational objectives, they can more effectively design appropriate learning strategies—and then attain the most desired learning level. Let's briefly consider the six learning levels.

- *Knowledge.* Level one emphasizes the ability to recognize and recall basic facts, technical terms, ideas, and phenomena.
- *Comprehension.* Level two requires the ability to understand information, to see interrelationships between and among concepts, and to use knowledge in some meaningful way.
- *Application.* Level three emphasizes the ability to apply knowledge appropriately and correctly and to develop problem-solving skills and approaches.
- *Analysis.* Level four requires the ability to break material down into constituent parts and then recognize the relationships (connections and interactions) between and among the elements.
- *Synthesis.* Level five requires the ability to combine (or recombine) elements in ways that form new patterns or structures and that lead to creative problem-solving and artistic activities.
- *Evaluation.* Level six emphasizes the ability to make judgments about the value of ideas, methods, and activities.

Each learning level requires the skills and abilities acquired in the preceding level. Through applying the levels of learning concept, both teachers and students can optimize the educational experience by first establishing their educational objective—and then selecting strategies that will best help them attain their desired objective.

Toward a new educational model

The knowledge explosion in recent years has presented medical education with large questions. How much do future physicians need to know? How should they learn? And how should they use what they learn? The Robert Wood Johnson Foundation has proposed some approaches to medical school education that ask all faculties and student populations to examine established attitudes and beliefs and to consider fresh perspectives and new educational strategies.[18]

Toward a New Educational Model

From: Traditional Model	To: Proposed Model
Comprehensive mastery of basic knowledge two-year pre-clinical curriculum	Selective mastery of only substantive foundation knowledge—six to eight month curriculum
Acquisition of memorized knowledge bank	Understanding of biopsychosocial and behavioral principles
Subject-centered with faculty dominant authority role and student in passive role	Student-centered with in faculty and students in learning partnership
Directed teaching/learning/ lectures that correspond with detailed syllabi of existing knowledge base	Problem-based, small-group, interactive discussions that address constantly a changing knowledge base
Discipline-oriented, step block teaching by autonomous departments.	Integrated, interdisciplinary teaching that crosses departments

Clinical applications presented after acquisition of basic science knowledge foundation	Clinical relevance and exposure to case material presented in graded detail from beginning
Emphasis on human biology and clinical skills	Emphasis on human development and growth
Training directed toward somatogenic illness, diagnosis, and cure issues	Training directed toward diagnosis and cure issues but with prevention and community orientation
Patient seen as passive object	Patient seen as partner in health transaction.

These suggested medical school curriculum changes reflect new scholarship and learning perspectives. And they suggest some ways medical educators can apply new educational principles and techniques to medical teaching activities. Moreover, the suggested changes reflect a growing humanistic emphasis and the need to see health and health care within a *social context*.

Toward a social perspective

Modern medicine continues to be dominated by the biomedical model—an approach to diagnosis and treatment that regards disease as a constellation of specific biochemical, physiological, and pathological anomalies—and that seeks mainly to relieve pain, prevent disability, and postpone death. Over the past 50 years, the biomedical model has made enormous contributions to our understanding of health and disease. But the model has tended to slight psychological, social, and behavioral influences—and to overlook the ways illness must be understood within the context of the patient's life story and continuing life experience.

In recent years, however, many clinicians, educators, and analysts (increasingly convinced that the biomedical model too narrowly interprets medicine's roles, functions, and tasks) have moved toward the *biopsychosocial model*—an approach that seeks to broaden the search for information and to move beyond the biological realm. The biopsychosocial model, the leading contender to succeed the biomedical concept, urges physicians and other professionals to understand the everyday settings and circumstances in which their patients live and work. *And the model seeks to bring together the science and humanism domains in ways that embrace both the observational and relational modes.*

George Engel puts it this way:

> By tradition the observational mode . . . is accorded scientific status, while the relational mode, as dialogue, is not. Yet in clinical practice, the physician always operates in both modes at the same time, making observations while engaging in dialogue and vice versa. The two processes thus not only are complementary and supplementary with respect to the results achieved, they are also interdependent in operation.
>
> The two modes address quite different categories of data and with different criteria. The observational mode is suited for phenomena that can be observed with the manifest behavior, the heart rate, or the level of serum bilirubin. . . . In contrast, a relational mode is required to deal with data in the uniquely human realm of articulated language, symbols, thoughts, and feelings by means of which what we privately experience is organized and communicated and relationships established and managed.[19]

Dr. Engel's admirable efforts to resolve some of medicine's humanism-science dichotomy—and to push medicine toward a broader biopsychosocial perspective—deserve our support. In today's brave new health care world, however, many analysts and planners have sought to push (or lead) medicine into an even broader perspective—into a paradigm that sees health care in its *social context* and that attempts to reorder responsibilities for true health.

Toward a social context of health

American society (and most societies) generally define health as the absence of disease. And Americans have structured a technologically-sophisticated, scientifically-oriented health care system that superbly *treats* specific illnesses and "critical incidents"—and that works mainly to contain the problem at hand. We value highly our medical care system, and we pour enormous resources into it—even though the main health status determinants seem now to lie beyond medical science's reach.

Over the past couple of decades, health planners and other analysts have trained increasing attention on the social context of health—on the view 1) that overall health status is largely determined by social environmental factors and 2) that true health consists of the ability to grow, develop, create, and change within a healthy and supportive environment. Social context advocates support medicine's traditional treatment interventions and applaud its ability to relieve pain and suffering. But they urge us also to consider the social determinants of health—and to address the psychological, physical, and social environmental elements that nurture and sustain health.

Health in this social context view, then, takes on a larger meaning. Good health in this broader perspective requires the opportunity to grow and develop within healthy family and community environments. And it demands the coordinated and synchronous contributions of all our domestic institutions—educational, economic, political, religious, civic, and medical. When we view health in terms of growth, creativity, and change, we begin to see the critical need for new research, educational, and clinical service agendas that will help us not only limit environmental assaults *but also foster healthy family and community systems.*

Can we finally identify the social determinants of health—and then adopt approaches to health and health care that integrate individual, family, community, and social perspectives? Can academic medicine find ways to explore the interrelations between and among various systems—and then identify important linkages? Perhaps a *systems perspective* can help us define the social context—and then draw boundaries around domains we can intellectually grasp and effectively change.

Toward a systems perspective

The health care system—broadly conceived—can be viewed as set of overlapping, interrelated, interdependent *systems* that seek (ideally) to develop each citizen's fullest physical, mental, and spiritual potential.

At the individual level, good health requires the synchronous, balanced, and integrated function of various organ systems. And medical practitioners spend vast amounts of time and resources attempting to keep the body's systems in balance—in a state of homeostasis. Modern medicine has developed a huge body of knowledge around these systems, and medical science continues to focus its main research activities on the function and care of individual systems.

Individuals, however, also possess psychological traits (and various belief and value systems) that directly affect health—for better or worse—and that strongly shape lifestyles, attitudes toward illness, and perceived health care needs. Practitioners attempting to see (and treat) the "whole person" must consider *all* the influences that impede or enhance health and development. And this holistic approach necessarily includes an examination of the family system, the community system, and the social system. Moreover, effective analysis requires the ability to identify a system's boundaries and to recognize the interrelations within, between, and among systems.

The family system especially influences individual health. And family values and mores strongly influence lifestyles and attitudes toward health and health services. In recent years, social analysts have trained increasing attention on the nature and function of family and community systems—and their relation to individual and social health. Universities and colleges have developed family medicine and family social science departments that examine family influences on health and illness. And the health care system generally accepts the view that healthy families enhance individual health—and that troubled and unhealthy families diminish health.

Individuals and families, however, also reside within community systems—within networks of medical, political, economic, educational, religious, judicial, and civic organizations that daily influence health and development. This community system supports individual and family health. And it links us to the larger social systems—a critical role in providing a sense of *connectedness*.

The medical and health care system largely conducts its activities within specific communities. And the community context offers academic medicine the richest opportunities for exercising the scholarly functions of *service* and *application*. In the words of Rudolf Virchow (written in 1849), "Should medicine ever fulfill its great ends, it must enter into the larger political and social life of our time; it must indicate the barriers which obstruct the normal completion of the life cycle and remove them. Should this ever come to pass, medicine, whatever it may then be, will become the common good of all."[20]

Academic medicine's increased involvement in the "larger political and social life of our time" hinges not only on a broader definition of scholarship—but also on a broader concept of health. This broader view sees health as more than the absence of disease. It seeks the fullest development of all citizens, and it strives to develop supportive family and community environments that enhance both individual well-being *and* the common good. And the challenge to academic medicine seems clear. In the words of Ernest Boyer:

> We need scholars who not only skillfully explore the frontiers of knowledge, but also integrate ideas, connect thought to action, and inspire students. The very complexity of modern life requires more, not less, information; more, not less, participation. If the nation's colleges and universities cannot help students see beyond themselves and better understand the interdependent nature of our world, each new generation's capacity to live responsibly will be dangerously diminished.
>
> This point, properly understood, warns against making too great a distinction between careerism and the liberal arts, between self-benefit and service. The aim of education is not only to prepare students for productive careers, but also to enable them to live lives of dignity and purpose; not only to generate new knowledge, but to channel that knowledge to humane ends; not merely to study government, but to help shape a citizenry that can promote the public good. Thus, higher education's vision must be widened if the nation is to be rescued from problems that threaten to diminish permanently the quality of life.[21]

The Chinese character for the term *crisis* consists of two characters—one signifying *danger* and the other *opportunity*. As medical educators decide how to direct their modern enterprise, they must hold in mind that medical education finds itself at the confluence of three forces: the *medical sciences*, the *medical profession*, and the *modern society*. The interests of these forces have remained remarkably similar over the years, and medical educators today face a unique opportunity: to give form to the inner logic of these convergent interests while pursuing a medical vision that will meet our medical needs.

REFERENCES

1. From "New England's First Fruits," a description of the founding of Harvard College, in David B. Tyack, ed., *Turning Points in American Educational History* (New York: John Wiley & Sons, 1967), 2.

2. Robert Wood Johnson Foundation, *Medical Education in Transition*, ed. Robert Marston and Roseann Jones (Princeton NJ: Robert Wood Johnson Foundation, 1992).

3. Leonard Duhl, *Health Planning and Social Change* (New York: Human Sciences Press, 1986), 141.

4. Ernest Boyer, *Scholarship Reconsidered: Priorities of the Professoriate* (Princeton NJ: Carnegie Foundation for the Advancement of Teaching, 1990).

5. Theodore Benditt, "The Research Demands of Teaching in Modern Higher Education," in *Morality, Responsibility, and the University: Studies in Academic Ethics*, ed. Steven M. Cahn (Philadelphia: Temple University Press, 1990), 94.

6. David Starr Jordan, *The Voice of the Scholar*, in Laurence Veysey, *The Emergence of the American University* (Chicago: The University of Chicago Press, 1965), 61.

7. Charles Eliot, *University Administration*, in Laurence Veysey, *The Emergence of the American University* (Chicago: The University of Chicago Press, 1965), 119.

8. William Bowen, *Ever the Teacher: William G. Bowen's Writings as President of Princeton* (Princeton NJ: Princeton University Press, 1987), 269.

9. Mark Van Doren, *Liberal Education* (Boston: Beacon Press, 1959), 115.

10. Clifford Geertz, "Blurred Genres: The Refiguration of Social Thought," *The American Scholar* (Spring 1980): 165–66.

11. Christopher Jencks and David Reisman, *The Academic Revolution* (Garden City NY: Doubleday, 1968), 252.

12. Oscar Handlin, "Epilogues—Continuities," in Derek Bok, *Universities and the Future of America* (Durham NC: Duke University Press, 1990), 103.

13. Jencks and Reisman, *The Academic Revolution*, 931–32.

14. Lee Knefelkamp, "Seasons of Academic Life," *Liberal Education* 76 (May-June 1990): 4.

15. Derek Bok, *Universities and the Future of America* (Durham NC: Duke University Press, 1990), 105.

16. Malcolm Knowles, *Self-Directed Learning: A Guide for Learners and Teachers* (New York: Association Press, 1975), 18.

17. Benjamin Bloom, *Taxonomy of Educational Objectives* (New York: Longman, 1986).

18. Robert Wood Johnson Foundation, *Medical Education in Transition*.

19. George Engel, "How Much Longer Must Medicine's Science Be Bound by a Seventeenth Century World View," *Family Systems Medicine* 10 (1992): 333–46.
20. Rudolf Virchow, in *Collected Essays on Public Health and Epidemiology*, ed. L. J. Rather (Canton MA: Science History Publications, 1985).
21. Boyer, *Scholarship Reconsidered: Priorities of the Professoriate*, 77–78.

SUGGESTED READINGS

Ernest Boyer, *Scholarship Reconsidered: Priorities of the Professoriate* (Princeton NJ: Carnegie Foundation for the Advancement of Teaching, 1990).

The Carnegie Foundation for the Advancement of Teaching, *Campus Life: In Search of Community* (Lawrenceville NJ: Princeton University Press, 1990).

Robert Wood Johnson Foundation, *Medical Education in Transition*, ed. Robert Marston and Roseann Jones (Princeton NJ: Robert Wood Johnson Foundation, 1992).

Roger G. Baldwin, "Faculty Career Stages and Implications for Professional Development," in *Enhancing Faculty Careers: Strategies for Development and Rewewal*, ed. Jack Schuster and Daniel Wheeler and Associates (San Francisco: Jossey-Bass, 1990).

Derek Bok, *Universities and the Future of America* (Durham NC: Duke University Press, 1990).

12

Inquiry and Change

The American health care system—a vast, fragmented array of services, programs, and organizations—stands at a crossroads. Powerful social, economic, political, medical, and scientific forces continue to drive policy decisions in ways that thwart coherent, deliberate problem-solving approaches. And American society continues to struggle with questions that go to the heart of some basic health care dilemmas. Questions, for example, like these:

- How can we balance our wish for freedom of choice and our need to maintain family health security?
- How can we balance our wish for fair health care allocations and our need to recognize the competing distributive justice principles of equality, equity, and need?
- How can we balance our wish for comprehensive, individual health care and our need to address the requirements of the common social good?
- How can we balance our wish for autonomous health care organizations and our need to develop an integrated health care system?
- How can we balance our wish for organizational flexibility and innovation and our need to maintain accountability and control mechanisms?
- How can we balance our wish for ethically acceptable decisions and our need to limit resources?

These questions—and others like them—reflect the cultural, social, institutional, and organizational *dilemmas* that underlie health care policy discussion and formulation. The dilemmas (defined by Webster as problems *seeming* to defy satisfactory solutions) perplex us—often confound us. But they needn't defeat us. Properly understood and viewed, they can help us frame health care issues in ways that promote change and innovation.

Social dilemmas

Many health care issues (access, quality, cost) lie rooted in a basic *social dilemma*—in a conflict between egoistic, self-serving desires and the requirements of the common social good. These dilemmas pervade social life and can be found at almost any level of social interaction. And our success in formulating viable health care reform proposals will rest heavily on our ability to understand and address these dilemmas—these conflicts between individual and common interests.

Individual interests operate powerfully—and they've been around for a while. In *Politics*, Book II, Chapter 3, Aristotle noted: "What is common to the greatest number gets the least amount of care. Men pay most attention to what is their own: they care less for what is common." More recently—in a 1968 *Science* article entitled "The Tragedy of the Commons"—Garrett Hardin illustrated the protypic social dilemma through a tale.

In Hardin's scenario, citizens of a small community are permitted to graze their cattle on the town's commons. The grazing costs are shared by the entire community, but each citizen is entitled to keep all proceeds from the sale of his or her cattle. Individual citizens gain by grazing additional cattle. But overgrazing destroys the entire commons and impoverishes all citizens—cattle owners and all others.

The cattle owners, pursuing unfettered self-interest, finally deplete the common resource and create a "tragedy of the commons"—an inevitable consequence, in Hardin's view, of unfettered freedom. "Each man," says Hardin, "is locked into a system that compels him to increase his herd without limit—in a world that is limited. Ruin is the destination toward which all men rush, each pursuing his own best interest in a society that believes in the freedom of the commons. Freedom in a commons brings ruin to all."[1]

Americans have held fiercely to a "frontier" mentality—to a view that more social resources lie "just beyond the horizon." As we approach the twenty-first century, however, we face some stark social realities. Infinite needs have collided with finite resources. And unchecked health expenditures threaten to deplete the other social institutions that nourish and support health and development.

In Garrett Hardin's view, only social and political solutions can resolve these "commons" predicaments. And he specifically recommends "mutual coercion, mutually agreed upon" approaches strategies we readily accept in certain areas of social life. Many "dilemma relevant" social sectors, however, resist "mutual coercion, mutually agreed upon" intrusions. And our health care system seems especially resistant to proposals that restrict individual freedoms. Meantime, however, powerful social, political, scientific, and economic forces continue to push change (and obstruct reform) in ways that leave little opportunity for broad discussion and debate—and little room for coherent, rational social problem-solving approaches.

Social dilemmas frequently intensify other already formidable obstacles to change. Various individuals and groups, for example, define the terms *solution* or *betterment* in quite different ways, and, consequently, often propose widely variant problem-solving approaches. Moreover, powerful interests (political, social, economic, and professional) have shaped and influenced each step in the health care system's development, and they have strengthened their positions with each evolutionary step. Although the system may resemble a "crazy quilt" at times, the underlying constellation of forces possesses a logical coherence, and these forces often work powerfully to maintain the status quo. Interest groups defend fiercely their ideologies, interests, beliefs, and values—and they resist invitations to *rethink* their value systems and conceptual frameworks.

Thus, social problem-solving in American society moves slowly—when it moves at all. And social reform often resembles (in Max Weber's words) "the slow drilling of hard boards"—an activity that many would-be reformers find ultimately unsatisfying.

In the face of all the daunting obstacles to change, a reader might wonder whether American society can formulate and institute *any* health care reform measure. Can we find any resolution to the seemingly intractable social, economic, and political dilemmas that impede health care system change? Can we extricate ourselves from the value conflicts and interest conflicts that paralyze decision-making—and then establish a process of *inquiry* that will foster true and lasting change?

We can and we must. First, however, we need to understand 1) that complex, interrelated health system forces resist change and 2) that approaches to change require a willingness to face complexities, to accept tradeoffs, and to examine continually the *value* conflicts and *interest* conflicts that underlie our social dilemmas. When we view dilemmas as consequences of value and interest conflicts, we begin to see opportunities for fundamental change. And we establish inquiries that allow all citizens ("experts" and "nonexperts") to aim at underlying values, beliefs, and attitudes.

Toward a civic health care voice

Over the years, we've tended to rely on various experts (so-called) for social change guidance. These modern social and natural scientists interact effectively with the new communications and computation technologies, and their *science-guided* problem-solving approaches have served us well. We can hardly imagine a world without them.

Yet, their investigative methods contain some inherent limitations. They rely heavily, for example, on empirical "proofs" and deductive reasoning, and they tend to stay well within their professional boundaries and academic disciplines. Moreover, they often slight the influence of constraining social and cultural values, and they tend to shrink from complex, "messy" social issues.

We've benefited from science-guided problem solving approaches, but along the way we've tended to discount (or at least overlook) the *self-guided* lay inquiry that directs us toward large existential, moral, and political questions. The science-guided model aims for conclusive answers. The self-guided (or lay probing) model, however, accepts inconclusiveness and assumes that certain social problems lie beyond the reach of conventional scientific approaches. And the model accepts a basic social reality: we tend to postpone social change until our distress reaches uncomfortable proportions—and until social conditions force us to reconsider the social, institutional, and political processes and values that block or limit change.

Thus, although empirical social scientific research can help us identify and isolate social problems, it cannot force a reconsideration of values and volitions. Only ordinary citizens, acting in concert, can move society toward a reconsideration of social values and a reformulation of social policies.

In recent years, the American public has grown increasingly distrustful of *empirical social science* and its ability to formulate effective social problem-solving approaches. At the same time, the public has developed a skeptical view of society's *ideological* rigidities, obfuscations, and imprecisions. And we now face critical questions. Can we develop an alternative to the *social scientific* and *ideological* problem-solving approaches that have left us with major unresolved health care issues? Can we develop processes of *inquiry* that will help us identify value conflicts and interest conflicts—and resultant dilemmas? Can we develop a social discourse that strengthens the decision-making voice of average citizens? And can we ultimately change our dispositions—our preferences, wants, needs, and interests.

Dispositions alter slowly, and some analysts argue for imposed solutions—designed and implemented by appropriate authorities. This authoritarian approach holds some appeal. But Americans tend to reject imposed solutions—even when the consequences are further inaction, stalemate, and deadlock.

Thus, when social scientific and political ideological solutions fail, the only viable choice (for both experts and common citizens) may be new *inquiries* into social attitudes and beliefs—a probing into the end-state and mode of conduct values that underlie our health care dilemmas. This broad inquiry or probing—an "unscientific" enterprise in the eyes of certain experts—invites individuals in many roles to participate in a dialogue (a "pool of common meaning") that defines dilemmas and formulates resolutions. And it holds out possibilities for incremental health care reform that may ultimately add up to meaningful system change.

Readers who have come this far will note that we've offered no broad policy proposals—no calls to "deregulate the health industry," or to "eliminate tax exemptions for health insurance," or to "introduce more competitive measures." Special interests and the cautious (and easily-blocked) legislative process resist measures that reorganize industries and economic sectors. And interrelated and mutually reinforcing social, institutional, political, and economic forces work powerfully to maintain the system's configurations and culture.

In this book, we've defined another approach. Throughout the discussion, we've offered various perspectives and "windows" from which to view the health care system. We've posed certain value, justice, and ethics dilemmas that seem to impede reform. And we've proposed new organizational, leadership, and educational models that we hope will move us toward more efficient and effective care systems. We'd like to end by offering a few conclusions (or discussion points) that illustrate the kinds of issues and dilemmas we think deserve inquiry—and that we hope will draw providers, policy makers, public officials, and average citizens into a richer and more *value-based* dialogue.

SOCIAL, SYSTEMIC, AND ORGANIZATIONAL ISSUES

Conclusion 1: *The social environment influences health status.*

Optimal individual health rests heavily on personal lifestyles and choices. But individual and collective health also rests on our ability to "manage the commons" and to create and sustain health-enhancing social environments. Socioenvironmental factors powerfully influence individual health and development. Environmental assaults and deteriorating suboptimal community environments impede physical, emotional, psychological, and spiritual development—and undermine individual, family, and community health. Some researchers now estimate that medical treatments account for only one-quarter to one-third of our overall health status. The other three-quarters to two-thirds, they say, can be attributed to poor lifestyle factors and social environments.

We've tended over the years to equate *health* with *health care*, and we rely heavily on the medical care system for help in defining and addressing our "health care needs." Over the past half-century, we've constructed a powerful *medical care model* that strives mightily to meet our health care wants and needs—and that provides remarkable (often miraculous) forms of care. We've developed great confidence in the medical model's ability to restore function and well-being. And the model continues to dominate health care and health planning activities.

In recent decades, however, we've increasingly turned to the medical care model for help in treating the consequences of *social ills*—unemployment, inadequate education, unsafe homes, and dangerous neighborhoods, for example. The medical system has responded well (often heroically) to these contemporary demands. But increasingly-prevalent socially-induced traumas, illnesses, and breakdowns now strain the medical care system's resources—and threaten to deplete other social resources that support health and well-being.

We've yet to place the medical care model into a larger health care model—and then understand the ways socioenvironmental factors (economic, political, cultural) influence health status. We continue to focus on the medical consequences of social ills—and to slight the development of an integrated social policy that prevents social breakdown and resultant health care problems.

Conclusion 2: *Health care organizations, programs, and services reside within a complex health care system.*

A health care organization represents a specific, boundaried system that contains various interrelated processes. That system interacts with other related systems—all of which reside within a total health care system. The total system—a complex array of programs and services—challenges our ability to see it whole. Systems thinking, however, allows us to define manageable systems around which we can draw boundaries and within which we can effect change.

When we adopt the *systems* perspective we begin to see "ripple effects" and "reciprocal flows of influence." We move away from the linear ("cause and effect") thinking that often freezes problem-solving approaches. And we begin to see that the pieces of our social organisms are independent yet joined, separate yet interconnected. Systems thinking improves our ability to understand the intrarelations within organizations and the interrelations between and among organizations, programs, and services—and it helps us enhance efficiency and effectiveness throughout the entire care continuum.

When stakeholders work with the movement and flow of simultaneous events within a familiar system, they learn that changes in small, well-defined systems build on each other—and hold the potential for creating large-system changes. By drawing boundaries around manageable and understandable systems—and then applying the most effective interventions at the most appropriate leverage points—stakeholders learn that little by little, system by system, they can create changes they never imagined in places they never considered.

Conclusion 3: *Significant changes in the health care system will occur at the organizational level.*

Health care services are delivered through a complex, interrelated set of health care organizations. And most health care change activities will occur within an organizational context. The Total Quality Management (TQM) approach offers large opportunities for establishing a culture open to change and capable of managing change. And a continuous quality improvement culture can help all organizational members see quality in terms of 1) internal and external customer *perceptions* and 2) efficient and effective interrelated *processes*.

The continuous quality improvement approach, striving always to reduce output variation, leans heavily on the W. Edwards Deming management philosophy and its Fourteen Points:

Point 1: Create constancy of purpose for improvement of product and service.
Point 2: Adopt the new philosophy.
Point 3: Cease dependence on mass inspection.
Point 4: End the practice of awarding business on the basis of price tag alone.
Point 5: Improve constantly and forever the system of production and service.
Point 6: Institute training.
Point 7: Adopt and institute leadership.

Point 8:   Drive out fear.

Point 9:   Break down barriers between staff areas.

Point 10:   Eliminate slogans, exhortations, and targets for
            the work force.

Point 11:   Eliminate numerical quotas.

Point 12:   Remove barriers that rob people of pride of
            workmanship.

Point 13:   Institute a vigorous program of education and
            retraining.

Point 14:   Take action to accomplish the transformation.

These Fourteen Points, together with Peter Senge's Five Learning Disciplines (*personal mastery, mental models, shared vision, team learning, and systems thinking*), form a "learning organization" culture that values employees, customers, and suppliers—and that simultaneously promotes individual growth and organizational development.

MEDICAL DECISION MAKING ISSUES

Conclusion 4: *The goal of health care is to maintain function.*

The acute care system—a complex network of caregivers, hospitals, and clinics—seeks largely to diagnose and *cure* specific illnesses. And we rely heavily on this system's ability to address illness and relieve suffering. Acute care patients and physicians, however, intent on cure, often fail to consider *function*—the ability to conduct desired activities of daily living in a chosen environment. And patients and physicians may at times pursue diagnoses and treatments that offer little (if any) prospect for improving the ability to participate in family and community life.

The chronic care system, on the other hand, dealing daily with multiple chronic diseases and inevitable decline, considers more carefully the ways interventions help maintain a patient's function—or at least slow its decline. Both systems provide invaluable care, but their differing focuses and goals interfere at times with their ability to provide integrated health care across the continuum.

The two systems, however, remain highly interdependent. And physician-leaders who understand the interconnections and inter-organizational linkages between them will enhance efficiency and effectiveness across the entire care continuum. Health care organizations and caregivers who consider both cure *and* function will improve quality of life—and perhaps even conserve resources.

Conclusion 5: *Medical interventions provide benefits and impose burdens.*

Medical treatments cure illnesses and restore function—and daily help citizens resume normal activities These medical interventions, however, also impose burdens. And in recent years, the benefit-burden issue has come under increasing scrutiny at both the individual and social level.

At the micro level, patients and families seek specific diagnoses and treatments—interventions that hold the prospect for improving a condition, worsening a condition, or creating a new condition. All medical interventions, however, impose some burden—some degree of pain and suffering or economic hardship. We readily and wisely accept treatment's accompanying burdens when the benefit seems clear and the risk low. Our expectations for cure, however, sometimes push us toward treatments that offer little benefit—and that may impose a large economic burden.

Physicians (and other caregivers) also seek cures and the best possible outcomes. Their humanitarian temperaments and professional natures (together with their desires to meet patients' expectations) often propel them to use the full diagnostic and treatment arsenal. And needed benefit-burden discussions sometimes get lost in the quest for cure.

Thus, various forces in the practice setting can merge in ways that obstruct (often defeat) careful consideration of potential benefits and burdens. In the pursuit of cure, patients and physicians may undertake treatments that offer little benefit and that carry high risk for imposing physical, psychological, and financial burdens.

At the macro level, the benefit-burden issue carries large economic and social implications. And it poses a classic social dilemma question: What is the balance between individual and group interests? Can we, for example, continue to provide expensive heart transplantation and renal dialysis programs (that aid a few) at the expense of prenatal and vaccination programs (that aid the many)?

Moreover, unchecked health expenditures threaten to deplete and erode the other social institutions that nourish individual and social well-being. And all citizens now must consider the ways specific health expenditures affect overall social well-being. We've begun developing some criteria for allocating care. And closer and continuing examination of the benefit-burden issue (at all levels) may improve our health care allocation decisions.

Conclusion 6: *Practitioners and patients strive for medical certainties in a health care system that deals in medical probabilities.*

We seek medical certainty in a health care world that offers only medical probability. And this zealous pursuit of medical certainty—together with high (often unrealistic) expectations for cure—clouds medical judgments, fuels costs, and threatens to deplete social resources that foster overall well-being.

The quest for certainty derives in part from our seeming unlimited faith in scientific medicine's curative powers. We relentlessly pursue causal explanations and "cures at all costs." Anxious patients, shielded by third-party payers, seek diagnostic and treatment packages that maximize certainty and minimize probability. And, in the face of illness and injury, patients rarely question recommended (albeit risky) technological "fixes"—and they seldom consider social costs.

Physicians, motivated by their humanitarian natures and commitment to the Hippocratic Oath, also seek the best possible outcome—usually defined as cure. And they, too, rarely consider social costs in the ordinary course of their diagnostic and treatment activities. Their strong scientific and technological orientation steers them toward reductionist approaches and causal explanations. And their reliance on technological solutions—together with a litigious environment that fuels a "defensive medicine" approach—drives costs and inhibits certainty-probability discussions.

Some medical ethicists reject any challenges to a totally patient-centered ethic. In Robert Veatch's view, any social cost consideration requires physicians "to remove the Hippocratic Oath from their waiting room walls and replace it with a sign that reads *'Warning all ye who enter here. I will generally work for your rights and welfare, but if benefits to you are marginal and costs are great, I will abandon you in order to protect society.'* "[2]

In today's harsh economic health care world, however, a totally patient-centered ethic and an unrestrained quest for certainty carries broad social implications. We face the *aggregation problem*—a dilemma that poses some serious questions. How much certainty can we afford? Can we develop decision-making tools that will enable us to make peace with uncertainty and still allow resource conservationa? And can we develop a communitarian bioethics that balances individual medical care interests against the exigencies of the common good?

Full and free discussion of the certainty-probability issue may help physicians and patients avoid diagnostic and treatment overkill—and may help society develop wiser health care allocation criteria.

ALLOCATION ISSUES

Conclusion 7: *Finite resources force consideration of medical care rights and limits.*

Policy analysts, planners, and public figures (of various political stripes) regularly decry our soaring health care costs—and for good reason. Infinite health care wants and needs have collided with finite resources, and American society faces difficult choices. Over the past 30 years, health care costs have exceeded overall economic growth in every year but three. And there's no end in sight. These exploding costs threaten not only the health care system but also the other social institutions that support health and development.

Cost-containment plans abound, and certain control measures have checked expenditures. We've yet, however, to address some central cost-control questions. Do citizens, for example, possess a right to health care—and, if so, to how much and what kind? Is health care a social good to be distributed according to need? Or is it largely a commodity to be governed by market forces? Or is it some of both? Should we impose limits—and if so, what kind? And who will decide?

When we characterize health care as a claim "right"—an absolute, guaranteed, individual right—we insulate it from competing resource claims, and we restrict care limit discussions. When we place health care in a social context, however, we see more clearly the social costs of unrestrained spending—and the need to develop ethical principles that will support reasonable treatment limits.

Our wants have become needs—and our needs have become rights. And cost-constraint proposals must take into account the ways we define health care goals—and whether we consider health care a freedom right or a claim right.

Conclusion 8: *Equity, equality, and need distributive justice principles conflict and compete.*

Distributive justice principles greatly influence our health care resource allocation decisions. They determine who gets what—and how much. And the principles frequently conflict and compete. Should society, for example, allocate health care services *equally* to all citizens? Or according to *need*? Or according to the *equity* principle—the ability to pay? Or according (most likely) to some combination of each? Our cost containment efforts—indeed, the level of our individual and social well-being—will rest heavily on our ability to balance competing distributive justice principles and to determine fair allocation criteria.

Distributive justice issues pervade medical life, and allocation decisions are finally grounded in definitions of health and health care. Is health care a *special* social good that stands outside the usual allocation considerations. Is it a basic social right? Or is it a market commodity? Or is it some of each?

Moreover, allocation decisions are also rooted in basic conceptual frameworks. When we support the medical model, for example, we strive for cure (the model's controlling metaphor), and we tend to slight social costs. When we move toward the larger health care model, however, we begin to see socioenvironmental influences, and we begin to think in terms of environments, systems, networks, interrelated institutions—and their contribution to health and development.

Thus, allocation decisions are determined not only by distributive justice principles but also by the conceptual framework in which we place medicine and health care. Close consideration of both will move us toward a more just health care world.

Conclusion 9: *The right to health care imposes responsibilities on both society and the individual.*

Medical care occupies a unique position in American life (and most other societies). Illness threatens our humanity and pushes aside most other considerations. And although we may continue to regard life, liberty, and justice as "absolute" rights, they cannot be exercised fully in the presence of injury and illness. Thus, although health care may remain a relative right in most regards, it also remains a moral imperative. And in our professed civilized, democratic, and humane civilization, we generally expect society to provide—even absolutely guarantee—needed medical care.

Does the demand for a right to medical care, however, assume reciprocal obligations—and does it entail certain restraints on individual freedom? If society guarantees the right to health care (in some general form), can it then expect citizens to assume personal responsibility for their health and well-being? At the policy level, we find it difficult to draw the line between encouragement and coercion. And Americans resist broad social problem-solving approaches that subordinate individual rights to the collective will and the interests of the common good.

Meantime the basic social dilemma—the tension between individual rights (or license) and social needs—continues to stall reform efforts. And we continue to learn that liberty and rights (including the right to health care) are paid for in the currency of obligation and responsibility.

Conclusion

This brief set of "conclusions" (the list could go on) illustrates the complexities underlying and surrounding basic health care issues. The observations, however, also illustrate some ways we can aim our inquiry at fundamental underlying causes and issues. Our health care dilemmas—rooted in conflicting conceptual frameworks, clashing values, and colliding interests—frustrate and confound us. But they needn't defeat us. If we can find ways to identify and analyze them, we may develop a broader (and calmer) dialogue. And we may ultimately constuct a more effective and humane health care system. We hope this book will provide some tools for establishing freer inquiry and a richer social discourse.

REFERENCES

1. Garrett Hardin, "The Tragedy of the Commons," *Science* 162 (1968): 124–48.
2. Robert Veatch, "DRGs and the Ethical Reallocation of Resources," *Hastings Center Report* 16 (1986): 32–40.

SUGGESTED READINGS

David Schroeder, ed., *Social Dilemmas: Perspectives on Individuals and Groups* (New York: Praeger Publishers, 1995).

Charles Lindblom, *Inquiry and Change: The Troubled Attempt to Understand and Shape Society* (New Haven: Yale University Press, 1990).

Garret Hardin and J. Baden, *Managing the Commons* (San Francisco: W. H. Freeman, 1977).

Lester Thurow, *The Future of Capitalism* (New York: William Morrow, 1996).

H. Margolis, *Selfishness, Altruism, and Rationality: A Theory of Social Choice* (Cambridge: Cambridge University Press, 1982).

Subject Index

Name Index

Aristotle
  on common good, 204
Alderfer, Clayton
  on needs (ERG theory), 27

Beauchamp, Thomas
  on rationing, 81
  on autonomy, 61
Bellah, Robert
  on rights, 48–49
Benditt, Theodore
  on education history, 184
Bennis, Warren
  on leadership, 158
  on power, 171–172
Berwick, Donald
  on quality improvement, 94
Blanchard, Kenneth
  on power, 172–173
Blank, Robert
  on unlimited care, 59
Bloom, Benjamin
  on levels of learning, 191–192
Bok, Derek
  on scholarship and society, 190
Bowen, William
  on research, 186

Boyer, Ernest
  on the function of scholarship,
    184–190
  on scholarship and the common
    good, 199
Burns, James MacGregor
  on leadership, 197

Callahan, Daniel
  on freedom and responsibility, 63
  on setting limits, 79–80
Childress, James
  on rationing, 81
  on autonomy, 61
Condorcet, J. M.
  on scientific medicine, 82–83

Deming, W. Edwards
  and total quality management,
    103–116
Donabedian, Avedis
  on quality, 92–94
Donley, Rosemary
  on ideological models, 73–76
Drucker, Peter
  on organizations, 88–89
  on the Knowledge Society, 88